WHEN BODIES BREAK

How we survive and thrive with illness and
disability

Cameron B. Auxer, M.A.

When Bodies Break: How We Survive and Thrive with Illness and Disability

Copyright © 2018, Cameron B. Auxer

To obtain permission to use material from this work, please email your request to Cameron Auxer at reader.writer@hotmail.com.

ISBN: 9781790541546

Imprint: Independently published

Dedication

This book is written in MEMORY of:
my father, William L. Auxer, Jr. (1926-2016),
my sister, Leslie Auxer (1956 - 2018)
and Angil Tarach-Ritchey (1960-2015);

in HONOR of:
friend, warrior and inspiration, Michael Fernandez and every
contributor in this book;

and DEDICATED to the billions of people worldwide who live with
chronic conditions and disabilities.

Table of Contents

PART 2 - How We Learned to Live Well with Chronic Illness and Disability

Chapter 1 The Devastation and Delight of Diagnosis

Chapter 2 Emotions, Changes and Suffering

Chapter 3 Self-Care and Creating Balance

Chapter 4 Becoming Your Own Best Health Care Advocate

Chapter 5 Your Passion, Your Purpose and Starting Over

Acknowledgements

Grateful acknowledgement goes to the many people who played a role in making this book possible.

Special thanks and big hugs to each contributor for your wholehearted belief in this project and for baring your souls to inspire and educate others. Through the years that we worked together, mostly online, you've become cherished friends to me.

My late father, William L. Auxer Jr, who bragged about my website to his friends, encouraged me along the way and bought me a new computer specifically for this book. Thank you, Dad! I only wish you were here to read this.

My late sister, Leslie Auxer, for gifting me with Microsoft Office. My angel, I couldn't have written the book without it. Oh, how I wish you could hold this in your hand.

Kari Ulrich, you held my hand (figuratively) when I was newly diagnosed with FMD and then became co-conspirator and mid-wife at the birth of my website. You have been generous with financial and moral support during this project. I am so very grateful, my sweet friend.

Anne Gaucher "Lyme Lens" (contributor, Chronic Lyme Disease fighter, photographer, blogger), for your proofreading and editorial assistance, and keeping your promises despite having to jump high hurdles with dicey health.

Writers Dallas and Joanne Barnes for your continued support. I'm blessed to have such excellent teachers and warm friends.

My fellow writers in The Write Way and Next Write writers' groups for your feedback and encouragement with this and other projects. You gave me the gift of confidence for which I am so very grateful.

My niece, Angelina Corrado, makeup artiste extraordinaire, and photographer, Michael Rose, both of Boston, for donating your services for my photo on this book's cover. Your talents are greatly appreciated.

Julie O'Connor for your artistic flair and willingness to interpret my ideas for the cover and translate them into a masterpiece! I bow in your presence!

Jennifer McKelvey Runyon for your assistance in polishing up the final draft and turning it into a self-published book.

My first BFF in childhood and beyond, Carole Donovan, for the design of the book cover. I also thank you for sharing with me the book, One Door Closes by Tom Ingrassia and Jared Chrudimsky. Not only was it inspiring but it also proved that the format planned for this book could actually work! Thank you for being there and believing in me for so many years.

To my friends with chronic illnesses, on- and off-line: amidst your worst sufferings, you are always there with an encouraging word for me. I will always be grateful

Introduction

Chronic illness has been a life-long companion on my meandering path. It wasn't until I experienced multiple heart attacks, leaving me chronically fatigued, and for several months without short-term memory, that life as I knew it stopped dead in its tracks.

These 360-degree turns in one's journey aren't necessarily all bad. They are great reminders to focus on self-care and offer wide-open doors to self-discovery. If I hadn't become as ill and depressed as I did, if I had not come to a complete stop at that point, I wouldn't have connected with amazing, inspiring, encouraging people on social media. I wouldn't have found the courage to create a website for people with chronic illness. I wouldn't have found the confidence to write this book. I made the best out of a bad situation and it all turned into a positive outcome! My new purpose in life became clear to me: help others with chronic illness to accept their limitations, embrace new possibilities and create a rich, joyful life.

I'd never written a book before, though I've been a writer for most of my life. I found the process daunting and wasn't sure if I was equipped for the task. I tip-toed into the possibility of creating a book chock full of good stuff for people like me, who had the carpet of life yanked right out from under them. Through the encouragement of my writing group and its facilitators, my confidence grew. An enthusiastic chronic illness community offering powerful stories, sound advice and support made the task less overwhelming and more meaningful. I embraced the challenge.

Having said that, it is truly a miracle that this book finally got published. During the submission process, many of the contributors became seriously ill; some were even hospitalized. Eventually, through literal blood, sweat and tears, the submissions poured in and I found myself with a pile of inspiring stories of courage, strength and survival. Incredible writers who suffer from chronic illnesses, rising like the Phoenix from the ashes, fought to submit their stories for this book, even when they struggled to rise out of bed at times. These stories aren't about being cured, though some folks have healed in various ways. Instead, these are tales of digging deep down into one's suffering soul and finding the guts to create a new life. A life with adjustments. A life lived with purpose. A life that works any way you can make it.

Then it was my turn: writing my contributions, editing others' submissions and organizing the material into a book. I was enjoying newfound energy after my chronic fatigue syndrome went into remission, so, piece of cake, right? The universe had other ideas for my well laid plans... So far, I had been able to juggle my life with caring for my elderly father and dedicating time to the book. However, on April 10, 2016, I was forced to turn my attention away from this book and become a fulltime caregiver.

A minor injury to Dad's hand then snowballed into sudden paralysis of his vocal cord and epiglottis (impacting his speech and swallowing), double pneumonia, seizures and the eventual diagnosis of metastatic cancer in his brain, creating the perfect storm of a healthcare nightmare. His health deteriorated rapidly. There were trips to and from the hospital and rehab, where medical mishaps, incompetence and neglect risked his life. He suffered needlessly for weeks and I had to fight like a mama grizzly bear for his protection. I finally pulled him out of rehab, took him home, hired professional caregivers to assist me and got hospice involved to make his last days as comfortable as possible. One and a half weeks later, on June 23, 2016, my father, William Lloyd Auxer, Jr., finally found peace.

My own peace was slow to come. After months of sorting out my father's affairs and his house, and dealing with enormous tsunamis of grief, I got back into the writing groove, despite a relapse with chronic fatigue. Just when I thought the book was going to come together, things got turned upside down yet again with new health issues and an unexpected eviction from my black mold-riddled apartment. Here we are, approximately three years after the commencement of this project, but finally this book is in your hands! **(Please read the Epilogue at the end of this book for the update of my personal story.)**

Perhaps it wasn't a miracle that got this book published, but <u>resilience</u>. Resilience springs from adversity so that we may survive and thrive. We may become bitter and angry, complain and throw in the towel. At some point, though, we get tired of mourning our loss of health and having things the way we want them. We take the giant leap forward to accommodate things we can't do and celebrate things we can! Everyone in this book has faced adversity to the point of wanting to throw in the towel. It is only through resilience that that these authors have their stories to share. Maybe one of these stories will help you hang on to your towel?

This two-part book was created in cooperation with 31 other resilient, chronically ill people with whom I have connected online. We've seen it all! Whether you are reeling from a recent diagnosis or have been chronically ill for years, you'll find inspiration in the stories in Part One of this book. These personal accounts are honest, sometimes raw, often painful and always inspiring. The backgrounds, illnesses and life experiences of the authors are diverse. The common thread between us is our resilience and commitment to creating a better life; gaining wisdom, insight and, sometimes, a greater sense of humor along the way. I hope our journeys will be an inspiration for you on yours!

In Part Two, we pool our experiences to support you in creating a new path in life. We share what we've learned to help you successfully navigate the medical system, become a health advocate for yourself and others, take better care of yourself, find your passion and create income, and deal with the emotions that come with life-changing events. Our desire is to help make your life easier, more purposeful and subsequently, more joyful!

Blessings to you on your chronic illness journey, my friend. I hope you have victories, big and small, and may you find joy on the road ahead.

Note: You will notice that the spelling in this book is not consistent. The contributing writers come from the USA, Canada, United Kingdom and Australia. I have tried to preserve the spelling style of each author, either British English or American English, and in editing, attempted to maintain their "voice," as well.

Disclaimer: *No information in this book should be used to replace professional medical care. Before trying anything new in your medical treatment plan, please consult your doctor.*

PART 1 - Our Stories

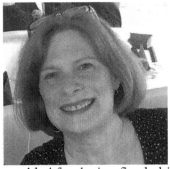

Cameron Auxer (USA)
Don't just survive, thrive!

My soul was determined to enter this world. After losing five babies, my mother was given Diethylstilbestrol (DES)* to avoid another miscarriage. I was born ahead of schedule, small yet hearty enough to go home.

My parents were heavy smokers, and I quickly developed asthma, multiple allergies and eczema and suffered frequent respiratory ailments keeping me home from school. As I grew, my legs often felt "loose" and painful and my stomach hurt at night. My hips would grind and hurt. Despite that, I still had fun being a kid and grew into a mischievous teenager.

I was thrilled to escape to college, enjoying my freedom, partying a lot and studying a little. I began nourishing my curiosity, creativity and sense of adventure, and hit my stride in my early adulthood with a career in radio. This also marked the beginning of my neck subluxations.

In the 80's, Kent State awarded me an MA in Speech Communication and Telecommunications; I was just shy of a doctorate when I walked away from academia. With my husband, I moved to Australia and became single soon thereafter, which is when I truly blossomed. I grew into a passionate traveler, visiting the jungles of Borneo and the outback of Australia, flying around the world more times than the first astronauts. I became a speaker, an environmental and human rights activist and a media producer.

Middle age dawned with excruciating migraines lasting up to eight days, severe dizzy spells and sometimes, both together. Thankfully, I lived in Australia when the migraine was at its worst, as the equivalent to Vicodin was available over-the-counter. Sadly, nothing helped with the dizziness and it was difficult to plan my life never knowing when these spells would hit.

I moved back to the US for a while, finding work in community health education and completing training in leadership and holistic health. Though my neck, shoulders and hips popped out causing pinched nerves, my back spasmed frequently and I suffered from osteoarthritis, asthma, migraines and dizzy spells, I remained active and energetic. Pain and illness had been my life-long norm but I chose to live a purposeful life!

New health issues started to emerge and snowball shortly after I returned to Australia and started working at a country boarding school. A hemorrhage in 2002 turned out to be uterine cancer requiring surgery (with a complication of internal bleeding). It was a frightening lonely time and the challenges didn't stop with the painful abdominal surgery. I went through a series of trials with hormone replacement therapy, some of which had no effect and some that caused allergic reactions.

After saving up enough money for tuition, I quit my job and began classes in naturopathic medicine. I had survived the hormone rollercoaster and did well until 2005, when heavy stress from several sources triggered three heart attacks over a period of eight days, during which one of my coronary arteries dissected. I lost my short-term memory for two months and collapsed into a period of chronic fatigue syndrome that would last ten years.

I had to withdraw from my studies and give up my dream of becoming a naturopath. To add insult to heartbreaking injury, I was forced off the hormone replacement therapy, which launched me abruptly into the flames of menopause. Nothing in my world felt right and it seemed like it never would. I waved a white flag at my conditions; I had had enough and couldn't compete with illness anymore. So began the toughest decade of my life.

My mother passed away a few months after my heart attacks, but as I was still healing and living in Australia, I couldn't visit my father until the following year. When I finally arrived in the States, I found an old man who was angry at the world and desperately in need of assistance. I flew back to Australia, sold or gave away most of my belongings, shipped the remainder of what little I owned to the US and boarded the plane with a heavy heart. I lost a piece of my soul as I left behind my close Australian friends, the loved ones I called family and the place I called home. What choice did I have? My dad needed me.

One week after moving in with Dad, I had heart attack number four. One month later, dad had one too, requiring a triple by-pass. I cared for him while I was still recovering and we eventually became the Father-Daughter duo at the Cardiac Rehab Center!

The cause of my heart attacks was determined to be Prinzmetal's angina (spasms in the coronary arteries). Treatment included long-lasting nitroglycerin which had the glorious side effect of triggering explosive migraines and did little to help my chest discomfort. My local cardiologist suggested I find a research hospital to better deal with my symptoms. I located a forward-thinking cardiologist and researcher who controlled the spasms with the amino acid, L-arginine.

This cardiologist also followed up on the noisy pulsations in my carotid arteries (bruits) which had been initially found by the doctor who did my exam for my Social Security Disability testing! An MRA (MRI with angiogram, showing the blood vessels with contrast dye) revealed carotids that resembled strings of beads and I was diagnosed with a rare, incurable disease called fibromuscular dysplasia (FMD). It took a while for the enormity of this diagnosis to sink in. How many doctors examined me and never caught this??

FMD can be found in any artery but most commonly in the carotid (neck leading to brain), vertebral (spine/neck leading to brain) and renal arteries. I have it in the carotids and vertebrals; in 2017, signs of FMD were also found in a mesenteric (sheath that lines the intestines bringing it blood flow) artery. The tell-tale sign of FMD is abnormal cell growth in an artery, causing it to twist or bead, often impeding the blood supply. In the carotids, where it is most serious for me, it can cause migraines and dizziness, and lead to aneurysms, dissections or stroke. FMD in renal arteries can affect blood pressure, leading to stroke. Research suggests that the disease may impact other connective tissue, as well, which may be why my tendons and joints have been problematic.

Eventually, I became a patient at the FMD program at Massachusetts General Hospital where I'm monitored by a team of exceptional doctors as part of their research. At this time, my condition is stable.

Perhaps having chronic illness as a child made accepting and overcoming limitations my norm. For most of my life, I just accepted horrifying medical news, got up, dusted myself off and soldiered on regardless of what I had just been told. It was like my outer layer was impenetrable. It wasn't until I was knocked down in mid-stride in my later years, stuck in bed or on a sofa or recliner, that I forgot how to get on with life and became challenged by the loss of my freedom and lifestyle. I threw myself one humungous pity party! I had to find a way back to how I used to manage adversity, chronic illness and bad news if I was going to survive and thrive.

What became integral in moving beyond my depression was remembering my strength and resilience and recognizing what I was able to do, as opposed to dwelling on what I couldn't. Connecting online with others who were chronically ill helped shift my perspective. As I healed my emotions, I became moved to help others who were ill to improve their lives. This became the mission of my website (pajamadaze.com), social media and this book.

In 2015, the chronic fatigue syndrome went into remission which, happily, allowed me to increase my activity level. Though chronic pain and illnesses continue to plague me as I age, and I get occasional CFS relapses, I am living more fully again. My adventures are more subdued these days and I must pace myself carefully. Despite this, I finally found my true joy: I became a wedding celebrant, which I love! What can be more joyous than joining two souls together on their journey through life? My life has become simpler, yet so much richer.

This is my promise to myself: though I know life can change abruptly with chronic illness, as long as I am able I will create each new day in a joyful way. If situations change for me, I will regroup and carry on. I will embrace the things I can do with as much zest and heart that I can muster. I will be good to myself. I will surround myself with love. Not only will I survive; as I continue on my journey in life, I WILL THRIVE!

(Please read the Epilogue at the end of this book for more of my story – this past year has been a doozy!)

Note: DES is now proven ineffective and impacts the health of mother and future generations.

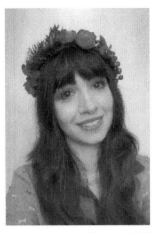

Ali West (UK)
Find sunshine on a cloudy day

I used to be a "normal" twenty-something with a good job as a lawyer and a busy social life. I went to the gym three times a week and had a boyfriend. Life was good. Then my friend lost her battle with cancer and it hit me hard. Months later, I was in the Dominican Republic for a wedding, when the anti-malarial tablets made me feel drugged. After that I was never right again.

I was back and forth with doctors over the following months. I felt totally exhausted; I'd come home from work and sleep. I suffered from severe headaches and panicked, thinking I had a brain tumour. My bloodwork was normal. Eventually, I was told I probably had myalgic encephalomyelitis (ME). I discovered a local specialist clinic and asked for a referral. It was there, in March 2003, that I was officially diagnosed.

I went through a mixture of emotions: relief at finally knowing the reason for feeling so poorly, but also sadness, as it meant my life would change. I pushed to keep working, as I didn't really understand the disease and didn't want to accept there was anything wrong.

I was referred to group therapy to help me learn to cope with this incurable disease. I was so newly diagnosed that I didn't realise how much it would affect me. I kept pushing myself until I collapsed. I took time off work, thinking I'd eventually be okay. After a few attempts to return to work, I had to accept that I couldn't continue.

We had just moved into our first home, living away from close family and friends, so I felt very isolated. I was practically bedbound and became depressed. I began taking various medications and after a while, started feeling more like 'me' again mentally but not physically. After twelve months, a meeting was arranged with my union rep. I wasn't well enough to attend and the decision was made that I couldn't return to work. It was almost a relief, despite losing everything for which I had worked so hard.

I eventually began to improve a bit physically and maintained a level of health for a while. During that time, my boyfriend and I got engaged, then married in Cyprus. I started struggling again, so was referred back to the ME clinic and an occupational therapist, as well as a psychiatrist to help me deal with accepting the illness. The clinic was helpful and I put some coping mechanisms into place. I learned that pacing myself by resting after every activity, no matter how small, does help. I also learned to challenge negative thoughts and not be hard on myself.

We decided to try for a baby and after ten months I became pregnant. My daughter was born in March 2009 – six years after my ME diagnosis. Within weeks after her birth, I suffered a relapse. I struggled and couldn't get through the days on my own, so my husband took some time off work. It was stressful but our beautiful baby girl was amazing! Thankfully, I was granted care through adult social services, which helped with things like food preparation and housework. That allowed my husband to work without worrying and me to look after my baby and rest regularly, knowing she was safe.

As my daughter got older things became slightly easier but my health never fully improved. She grew up sitting on my knee in my wheelchair that I use when we're out. Luckily, my care continued and though things were difficult, my daughter was happy and she brought much happiness to our lives. Once she started school in 2014, I started making bracelets when I felt up to it. I enjoyed creating and gifting them to friends and family, as well as making them for myself.

Soon word got out about my bracelets and what a lovely feeling it was to be asked to make them for others! I didn't feel useless or painful while I was creating. Having a distraction on which to focus made me happy. I started doing random acts of kindness, sending a bracelet with a card to make someone smile. I made some very good friends online, as well!

I appreciate the little things in life. I always laugh and find something good in each day, no matter how small. My advice to you is to listen to your body, don't push yourself, take time to accept the situation, then focus on what you enjoy that you CAN do! Find the sunshine on a cloudy day and remember, laughter is the absolute best medicine!

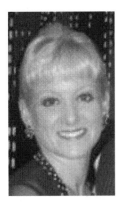

Anne Gaucher (USA)
Starting over, again and again

My life before chronic illness was fast-paced; always in the top of my class, always pushing for more. In my late teens and early twenties, I was a competitive figure skater training at the Olympic Figure Skating Arena in Lake Placid, New York. I went off to college and tried to keep skating but hit my first major roadblock in life: too many injuries, no financial supporters and I was getting too old. My dream of a career on the ice ended and I was devastated. It was time to start over.

I moved back to New Hampshire, working on a college degree part-time in Business Management and making a living as a bartender. While waiting on two EMS instructors, I was lucky enough to find my calling. They let me sit in on the EMS class the following night and I never looked back. I had a new passion in my life and it was full steam ahead!

I went through the three stages of training: EMT-Basic, EMT-Intermediate and then became a paramedic, all while working on an ambulance full-time. I also trained others to become EMT's, as well as teaching CPR and specialized programs. My favorite contribution to EMS was volunteering for my hometown Fire & Rescue Department. I was living my dream until I blew out my shoulder carrying a 400-pound patient who was having a heart attack, requiring three surgeries between 1999-2001, with each recovery lasting four-to-eight months. It was the end of this paramedic's career. Not only was I dealing with the shoulder, physical therapy, a worker's compensation battle and being out of work; this is when I was bitten by my tick (year 2000).

I had treated my cat for fleas and ticks, but she must have had a hitch hiker that night when she came in the house and curled up at the foot of my bed; the next morning, I found a HUGE engorged tick at my hairline! After rapid removal the proper way, I called the doctor, but was refused antibiotics, refused an appointment and refused a test for the tick. I had no symptoms of Lyme disease so, to him, I was negative. Period. (I wish he could see me now. Bastard.)

Time to start over again, first it was the end of skating and now I couldn't be a medic with a busted wing, eh? This time, graduate school to become a physician assistant. Flash ahead two years: just graduating, with a recurring sinus infection, despite three rounds of antibiotics. In three days' time, this became the worst headache of my life which advanced into aseptic meningitis in 2005. I had been looking for a job, under a lot of stress financially with student loans coming due soon and I was studying for the board exams, so my immune system was low. I wasn't even thinking about the tick. I rested for six days and got on a plane for job interviews in Florida.

I got through the Jacksonville and the Tallahassee interviews but had to give up and come home; the pain in my head was so bad I couldn't drive anymore. Worst plane trip of my life; I cried the whole way home. Turns out, I was leaking spinal fluid out of the spinal tap hole for 20 days since the tap for the meningitis and I needed an epidural blood patch to block the hole! It was done the morning after I landed, in the hospital recovery room next to the operating room. People couldn't believe that I had survived job interviews in that degree of pain. I told them, "When you want something badly enough, you can overcome anything."

I wanted the Jacksonville job, but was offered the Tallahassee job instead. *Screw it, I like Jacksonville, there are seven hospitals there and someone will hire me.* I sold my house in six days, packed or got rid of what wouldn't fit into a thirty-foot RV, tucked in my fourteen-year-old cat (I forgave him for the tick incident by then) with all my worldly goods and off we moved to Jacksonville, Florida, meningitis and all.

It's when I got to Florida that my health began to deteriorate significantly. I started my job doing in-patient critical care and even though I was working sixty to eighty hours a week, it was the best job a new grad could ask for! I was learning so much, I had complete autonomy and I had free reign of a 528-bed hospital. I LOVED my job almost as much as being a paramedic! I started competitive ballroom dancing and found the passion I had lost after being unable to skate. I had a life again but was tired all the time. I started to ache and the joints in my feet swelled if I danced too long. I knew there was something wrong.

I'd found a neurologist as I still had daily headaches from the meningitis. He did a spinal tap in 2006 (negative) and annual brain scans, but a spinal tap in 2007 was POSITIVE again. Something was VERY wrong: you don't get meningitis twice without cause. I saw fourteen doctors, but, finally, it was my research on the computer, and the suspicion of my primary care doctor in 2010 when my right wrist blew up, that found the culprit: "I think you have Lyme disease" were the words out of her mouth. I had completely forgotten about the gosh darn tick from 10 years ago. The crazy cat was still alive at 19 years old, on lasix for congestive heart failure but literally in better shape than I was.

My life changed completely. I lost weight 35 pounds on a petite 5'2" frame, then my cognition was gone. I was adding on my fingers (a woman with a Master's Degree, mind you), I lost my memory and then eventually it was time to leave my job. I had to fight to win my Disability. I was one of the lucky ones. Chronic Lyme disease is not recognized as a disease that people get disability for on their first time through the court system. Apparently, I was so sick that they called me on a Saturday morning to tell me that my request was granted immediately!

Dancing was too painful. I couldn't do housework and stopped driving due to balance issues, so I moved in with my mother. Things got bad quickly because I suffered from high vitamin D, as well. I received a multitude of treatments, one of which nearly killed me; I was going into bone marrow suppression, so all drugs were stopped. I was bedridden for three years, weighed 97 pounds, needed assistance to the bathroom and looked like a ninety-year-old. I developed a heart condition, dead adrenal system, thyroid condition, and was surviving POTS (postural orthostatic tachycardia syndrome, causing excessive tachycardia and other symptoms upon standing) with bags of fluid every day. Again, time to start over.

I was driven three hours each way to Melbourne Beach to see a chiropractor who also practiced applied kinesiology. In two years, he helped me regain my weight with supplements and testing and kept my disease at bay without antibiotics. I've slowly gotten stronger. I requested home physical therapy, have undergone hip surgery without complications and started outpatient physical therapy.

Right now, tachycardia remains the biggest stumbling block. I have survived thyroid problems and that is under control. Severe weight loss which is now stable. Tremors which have resolved. The memory issues are gone. Now I battle a heart rate at rest which is 110; if I walk to the car in the driveway it shoots up to 150 and I feel like passing out. The cardiologist is at a loss for a solution to what is going on, but you know what? It is just another opportunity to start over. I will not give up. This makes six years in bed now and I have had every treatment for this disease that exists on this planet. I will find another cardiologist and let him have a go at it. Someone somewhere will know how to slow down this heart rate so I can resume a normal life again. There will be a day when I can take a shower once again in hot water or eat a meal sitting at the table with my family and not being served a plate in my bed. I have been trapped in my bedroom for almost my entire 40's but that is OK because I am a patient woman.

I have lost EVERYTHING that was important to me. My career, my retirement money, my friends, my social life, my health, my hobbies, dancing, skating, my beautiful apartment in Riverside overlooking the river, money to survive on, even my beloved cat died, but I have the one thing that matters most to me: the love and support of my 24/7 caregiver, my mother who is still by my side in this crappy little apartment we had to move to because she said that she would never leave me. As sick as I have ever been, she has always been by my side. We may have nothing, but we will starve together. There is something to be said for the love shared between a mother and daughter. She is the reason that I will face every day and try to START OVER again and again and again.

You can read more about my story, my life and my viewpoints on my website at: www.lymelens.com.

I also share my photographs and love of photography on my blog at this website. Please feel free to write in and I will reply to your comments. It is my view of life through my Lyme Lens. Thank you for taking the time to read my story. I hope your journey has someone in it who encourages you to keep starting over and never give up.

Thank you to Cam for allowing me to proof this manuscript. I value her friendship dearly and her trust in me to handle her "baby" with the reverence that it deserves. This team effort has been a labor of love and I hope that it opens the eyes of the world to the masses of people out here who are suffering in silence with invisible illnesses.

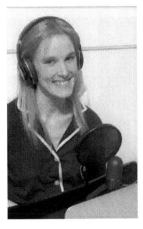

Rebecca Doss (USA)
Each day brings possibility and hope

I live in Kentucky, graduating with a degree in English in 2011. I enrolled in every creative writing course available in college to immerse myself in words and language. Words were my first love.

I married my other love, Roger, in June of 2011. The love of a loyal spouse is one of the greatest gifts in existence and I don't take it for granted. I thank God daily for giving me a partner who stays beside me unconditionally as we navigate life—and chronic illnesses—knowing God will deliver healing in His time.

Before chronic illnesses paused my life, I had many passions in addition to words, including figure skating, visiting family, attending church, and watching Kentucky Basketball with enthusiasm. I'm now unable to enjoy these activities due to diseases that ravage my body.

I was often sick as a child, and in ninth grade, developed anorexia and then a laundry list of diagnoses for seemingly unrelated issues, including obsessive-compulsive disorder, juvenile arthritis, trigeminal neuralgia, fibromyalgia, chronic fatigue syndrome, depression, anxiety, panic attacks and more. Nothing helped my symptoms and no doctor dug deep enough to uncover the underlying problems.

It took countless trips to specialists in Cleveland, New York City and other cities but we finally found the doctor who uncovered the real problem just two hours from home. In 2013, after quitting my job at age 24, we learned I'd been fighting chronic neurological Lyme disease and several co-infections and autoimmune disorders, since childhood. I started seeing my current doctor later that year, a caring Christian man through whom God is facilitating healing.

My symptoms used to be manageable; I could sit on the porch or cook an easy meal. On good days, we'd go to the movies, library or mall. I'm now bedridden with disabling pain and fatigue. Trigeminal neuralgia is called a "suicide disease" due to the severity of pain; mine is a byproduct of chronic autoimmune disorders. All traditional and non-traditional treatments have been or are deemed likely to be unsuccessful.

Roger is my caregiver in addition to his full-time job. He prepares meals, does daily tasks and carries me to the bathroom when I can't walk or crawl. I have difficulty understanding things I read and when speaking, I have trouble piecing thoughts together and communicating. Sometimes I forget my own name or how to spell it. I can't have visitors due to light, sound and smell sensitivities that create chaos in my nervous system.

My life was stolen by these diseases; they've taxed my physical, mental and spiritual strength. People say God gives his hardest battles to His strongest soldiers, but I remind myself that it's not my strength that keeps me going—it's my *knowledge* of God carrying me through this, even when I feel like giving up. That's what faith is: *knowing* something you don't see or feel.

With chronic illness comes loss. Good things also come with this journey; they're just harder to see amidst the struggles. I now appreciate things I used to take for granted. *Going from room to room with my walker? Opening my right eye? Having a conversation?* All things worth celebrating!

I wouldn't have found my calling if not for these illnesses. I've always loved Christian Hip-Hop, but never had the courage to record my own. In 2015, He spoke to my heart clearly, saying Christian Hip Hop must be a part of my ministry if I want to be an effective witness for Him. I'm recording an album right here from bed, hoping to encourage others, sharing truth, and giving glory to God, despite circumstances. Christian Hip Hop is one thing I can count on to keep my mind focused on God and not my problems. The joy brought by writing a lyric that resonates with others, or finding the perfect instrumental, is indescribable. That's proof enough God is always working, even if I don't *feel* it.

I urge anyone with chronic illness to not accept a vague diagnosis. Be persistent. Ask your doctor why you feel like you do, discuss underlying issues and ask what you can do to heal, instead of just manage, your symptoms. The chronic life isn't easy but fighting is not optional!

We're all pieces in the puzzle of humanity; while we can't see all the pieces or know what comes next, we must wake up and thank God for another day, struggles aside. Each day brings possibility and hope, even if it's hard to acknowledge those things, and our purpose is greater than we may ever know.

That's what keeps me going—the promise that one day the pieces *will* come together and, maybe, someone will find encouragement through the sharing of my journey on my website lymeislame.com. You can also find some of my music, along with others' music I enjoy, on soundcloud.com/grammaticallyso!

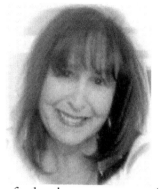

Abbie Levy (USA)
I am not my disease

For as long as I can remember my health was problematic. Having many missed days of school was my norm. Although I had good health care, the imaging we have today was not available back then. Not knowing what was wrong with me took quite an emotional toll through the years.

My three adult daughters have often told me what it was like growing up with an unpredictable mother. There were periods of time when I was living life to its fullest: enjoying my girls' activities, doing volunteer work, having friends for dinner. I enjoyed all the activities that most of us take for granted. There were also too many pajama days.

In my late twenties, my problems started getting some names. I was diagnosed with a congenital kidney disease called medullary sponge kidney. While this doesn't cause reduced kidney function, I had more bad kidney infections and kidney stones than I can count. I also began having severe inflammation and infection in my colon, which plagued me through my forties. Emergency rooms and overnight hospital stays became all too common.

My health problems took on a whole new meaning when a drooping right eye led to a diagnosis of an aneurysm. Fortunately, the aneurysm is small and is still being monitored. Six months after diagnosis, while reading a book in bed, I began to have stroke symptoms. I discovered that these symptoms were caused by a transient ischemic attack (TIA) or "mini-stroke." I was perplexed because I thought I had no risk factors for stroke.

After being discharged, I obtained my imaging report from the angiogram I had six months earlier. It was then that I learned that a vascular disease called fibromuscular dysplasia had been found. This disease, better known as FMD, was in both internal carotid arteries and both vertebral arteries. I also learned that the CT scan showed I had a previous stroke that affected my left frontal lobe. While I had been

19

having various neurological symptoms for many years, I can't say with any certainty when that stroke occurred.

As FMD is a rare disease, many doctors know little about it and there is no cure. Luckily, I found a website called Fibromuscular Dysplasia Society of America. There I found a wealth of information and discovered that aneurysms and stroke are two of the complications of carotid artery FMD. The disease also causes migraine-like headaches with which I have suffered for many years, as well as the whooshing in my ears.

After the TIA, the doctors also wanted to test me for a fairly common heart defect called patent foramen ovale (PFO). In some patients, a PFO can cause strokes. I tested positive. Within days I went from thinking I had no risk factors for stroke to learning I had two. The good news was the PFO could be repaired and was an easy procedure.

The saying, "Be careful of what you ask for!" applies well to my desire to have "names" for my numerous health issues. Ironically, by naming them I could begin to heal the emotional toll I had suffered for many years. As my Internist said, "Most all of your health issues are congenital. The writing was on the wall the day you were born." Wow, so this was not my fault; there was no one to blame!

Sometimes the difficult things in life lead to real gifts. The greatest gift I've received is the true meaning of acceptance, which has allowed me to be gentle with myself. I have also learned that "Knowledge is Power." Learning as much as I could about my issues has helped take the power away from the illness. I feel fortunate, now that I know what is going on in my body and can be followed by competent doctors. I've also found it helpful to join a wonderful support group for people with FMD. Helping the newly diagnosed gives me back far more than I give out.

Maybe the biggest gift of all was becoming my own advocate. This formerly passive woman now speaks up and takes an active role in her own health care. I have always lived life by the "Serenity Prayer," but it now has deeper meaning for me. Learning to accept that I can't change my health issues empowers me to change the things I can.

I am not my disease. I am "Me."

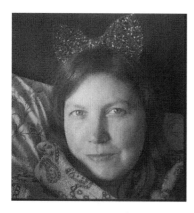

Charlotte Green (UK)
I feel more alive

In hindsight, there were early signs of illness years before I actually became unwell. Those symptoms were so mild that I didn't realise something was wrong and I was able to live a healthy, active life right up until my illness was triggered more severely.

I was a reception teacher for a class of 4- and 5-year-olds. While I loved working with my students, there were pressures outside of the classroom. The job became increasingly demanding as paperwork and procedures took time away from focusing on the children. In the summer of 2011, I married and took off on my honeymoon. The combined stress of a difficult year at work, organizing a wedding, getting vaccinated for my trip, long flights, followed by a week of bountiful food and alcohol, all took a toll on me.

Shortly after returning home, I came down with a virus causing a nasty infection in my chest and then my sinuses. Though both eventually went away with antibiotics, my body never fully recovered. I began to suffer body aches and pains, as well as swelling in my hands and feet. I tried carrying on with daily life but eventually my body gave up. Only able to lie in bed and sleep, I was signed off work. My doctor diagnosed post viral fatigue just before Christmas 2011. As I still hadn't recovered a year later, my diagnosis changed to myalgic encephalomyelitis, also known as chronic fatigue syndrome (ME/CFS).

My condition has fluctuated ever since. At first, I could go out for a couple of hours a day, with plenty of rest before and after. As is the case with many ME sufferers, I was told to push through the discomfort and that "exercise will cure you." Now I know that is exactly what you shouldn't do but I had followed the advice because I desperately wanted to get better. I became significantly more ill to the point of being bed-bound and unable to cope with any activity. All I could do was rest in a dark, quiet room.

Although supportive, my doctor has not given me much information about or help with my condition. Most of what I learn comes from the Internet or other ME sufferers. It was a scary, confusing and emotional time trying to get a handle on what was wrong and how best to recover.

There were many times in those early days when I didn't think I could carry on. Being in constant pain and not knowing what was wrong, or if you'll ever improve, is tough. With the help of my amazing husband, I got through that bleak period and learned to make the most of life, regardless of my limitations. It's lucky we had been together for 10 years before we got married; he loves me despite my ailing health!

The wonderful support network of chronically ill folk on social media has helped me come to terms with my new life. I've made some extremely close friendships, though I have yet to meet most of these people face-to-face. Through Twitter, I also got involved with Team Princess, a campaign to raise money and awareness for ME that allows sufferers to take part even if they're confined to bed. Every May 12th, we dress as princesses to highlight that, for us, there is no happy ending until a cure or treatment can be found. These virtual friends have also helped me understand my illness by swapping tips and experiences.

Now I can better manage my symptoms, allowing me to make gradual improvements and get back some quality of life. I've discovered what works best for my body. I've stopped listening to advice and instead, listen to my body. Acceptance of my illness and my limitations has been key to recovery.

It seems ironic but these days I feel happier than when I was healthy. I remain not well enough to work but I laugh more. I now appreciate every little aspect of life and enjoy the smallest activities. Worrying is a pointless waste of energy and will not change anything. Bitterness and anger, particularly regarding the bad medical advice I received, impacts negatively on my health. Similarly, fear achieves nothing other than holding you back from making the most of life. It saddens me to think about how insular I became when I first got ill.

I've learned that you never know unless you give it a go! Now I have the confidence to share my poetry and writing online and I sell my crafts and jewelry through a website for chronically ill crafters. Prior to my illness, I lacked the self-confidence to believe my efforts were worth sharing. I learned that failure is simply a part of life; it's how we learn, grow and improve. I find it quite poetic that it took failing health to teach me that. Despite the pain, the discomfort and the restrictions on my physical capabilities, I feel more alive now than I have in years.

Cindy Yee Kong (USA)
You're the one who must define yourself

I was born in Fuzhou, China and was a normal little girl until the age of eight when I suddenly showed symptoms of a mysterious disease that baffled my family and many doctors. I lost control of my body and when I lost that, I lost the sense of who I was. My body twitched, I couldn't speak clearly, slurring my words, and I had a learning disability. It was hard for me to go to school and to do what was expected of me at home. None of the doctors in Hong Kong could figure out what was wrong. Eventually, my mother and I immigrated to New York City to reconnect with the rest of the family; my father and my two older brothers.

I was eager to meet my father for the first time but this meeting turned out to be a dismal disappointment. My father was an alcoholic and physically abusive, never showing me any kind of love. My mother, who was illiterate and can't speak a word of English, wasn't able to get me proper medical help. My two older brothers wanted nothing to do with me. My father decided to stop supporting us financially, which drove my mother to work long hours in a sweatshop in Manhattan's Chinatown, earning meager money to put food on the table.

In the evening, I'd kneel and press my toes to the floor to do my homework which was one of the ways I managed the violent trembling and jerking so I could get my work done. It was a struggle. After homework, I bathed myself, washed my clothes by hand, made my dinner and got myself ready for bed.

A doctor who I trusted, sexually molested me. I became quite depressed and attempted suicide twice but was saved by Divine power. I realized there was a purpose for my life and went on a journey to find who this Divine being was. In high school, a friend introduced me to this God called Jesus Christ and I accepted Him as my Lord and Savior.

I worked hard in school and despite being learning-challenged in reading comprehension and the ability to understand oral information, I excelled academically and received honorary awards. Stories about my achievements were published in newspapers. During my last year of high school, I became a permanent resident of the United States which afforded me the opportunity to go to college.

One summer break, I was brutally attacked while on my way to work. I lived with fear and shame. I had learned from my home environment that I could only depend on myself, but it was difficult to deal with the pains of abuse, neglect and being an outcast. I endeavored to turn my pain into something positive; to help others by earning a sociology degree and become a social worker.

It wasn't until 1995, two years after college, that I received a proper diagnosis for my condition, dopa-responsive dystonia, a neurological disorder like Parkinson's. It took another decade for the rest of the mystery to unfold. When I eventually moved to Oklahoma, frustrated by my inability to maintain my job and relationship, I saw a speech pathologist and was diagnosed with central auditory processing disorder (CAPD). This condition stemmed from the original diagnosis of dopa-responsive dystonia. The speech pathologist told me that I can't process what I hear in the same way others do because my ears and brain don't fully coordinate. This means I have trouble hearing the difference between certain sounds. As a result, I may say 'dat' for that or 'free' for three. I'm easily distracted and have problems with reading.

I have difficulty articulating, speaking clearly and expressing myself with others. I also have limited facial expressions and voice inflection. I could be happy but sound like I'm yelling. When I'm stressed, I express a decrease in overall motor function and facial expressions, slurred speech, less understanding through what I hear and limited mobility.

In 2010, I was referred to a geneticist who confirmed my condition and this brought me to another level of understanding. The genetic testing revealed two recessive genes, each from both parents. My parents' children had a 25 percent chance of getting it. I was the unfortunate one. A mutated gene called tyrosine hydroxylase, which is critical in the production of dopamine, affected my movements, speech, learning, focus, displayed emotional behavior and flow of information in my brain.

25

The treatment for dopa-responsive dystonia is L-dopa. It helps to manage my uncontrollable twitching so I can coordinate my hands and feet and make my speech understandable. I suffered unfavorable side effects from the pharmaceutical medicine I was given so I switched to nutraceutical medicine under the supervision of Joel Robbins.

This condition makes it difficult to maintain relationships. I live with my husband and pets. I don't have many friends as it's difficult for me to keep afloat in conversations without having someone repeat, spell or draw out the words they're saying.

My main message to you is this: you're the one who must define yourself, not the medical profession, parents, friends, siblings or your disability. I wrote my book The Eyes of the Lion to help those struggling to keep moving forward and not give up.

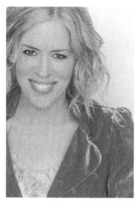

Cynthia Toussaint (USA)
My battle for grace

As a woman ravaged by intense pain and the loss of virtually all my life's goals, I have been transformed by suffering and love and brought to a higher place.

It all began in the 1980's when I was with the man I love, John Garrett, who is still in my life today. I was a 21-year-old ballerina with a bright future — one where I would dance, act and sing. The core of this was ballet—my greatest love and my identity since I was seven.

Ballet meant more to me than anything else. I didn't think anything could be more beautiful and there certainly wasn't anything that made me feel more whole. Growing up, I was always in leotards with my hair in a bun. In ballet, you're either right or you're wrong. I loved that structure and discipline. Nothing felt so good as the high of it, the sweat, putting that movement to the music. This was my absolute passion. Nothing was going to hold me back. Nothing.

Then it all came to an abrupt end. A minor ballet injury in my right leg triggered a chronic pain disease, complex regional pain syndrome, too often called "The Suicide Disease."

For thirteen years, the doctors said my problems were all in my head. I was left bedridden for a decade and unable to speak for five years while the CRPS spread throughout my body and attacked my vocal cords. During that time, most everyone in my life left me.

I was now just a young woman who used to be a ballerina. I had planned my entire life around performance. Then, in a moment, it was gone. At first, I wouldn't accept that I wasn't going to dance again. As the months and years ticked by, I watched others go on with their lives.

When I couldn't live in denial anymore, I became bitter, hateful, even suicidal. Wracked with anxiety, depression and waking with night terrors, I was lost. I was no one.

In those dark years, when anything negative happened, I raged, hurt myself, hurt John. I became a verbally and physically abusive person because I thought I had the right. After all, I was suffering, a victim who'd been cheated out of her life. I was drowning in self-righteousness.

I never imagined I might someday turn my suffering into something of value. In the mid 1990's, in ways I didn't understand at the time, I began making positive shifts in my life.

I knew I wanted to help others avoid what happened to me. I dropped the Cynthia-as-ballerina identity, a humungous shift, and began to reinvent myself. Finally and most importantly, I accepted suffering as an intimate part of me and, indeed, my new normal.

I found a voice as a healthcare reform advocate and launched "For Grace" to help other women with life-altering pain. But I was still searching for peace. I needed to purge and self-examine.

Writing <u>Battle for Grace</u>, John and I were given the opportunity to re-visit our traumas and suffering. For the first time, I saw a world that was bigger, by far, than the one I was born into.

As we wrote and read our story aloud, I saw up close the bad energy I'd created. As the words were carved out, I realized I could stop this chain of pain and violence.

Instead of resentment, I could practice appreciation. Instead of hate, I could enjoy love. Instead of blame, I could forgive.

I forgave the doctors who failed me, who told me I was crazy. I came to recognize that they did the best they could.

I no longer felt resentment for those who left me. They too were traumatized by my pain and the absence of any healing.

I befriended my disease and as I came to appreciate it as a part of who I am. I loved myself more deeply.

I also discovered new ways to enjoy more healing and better tomorrows.

The power of narrative therapy — in this case, writing our book — is a wondrous tool to re-examine our internal demons. That's why I urge fellow sufferers to use daily journal writing to help them connect the dots and open the doors to positive action.

Being comfortable with "what is" allowed me to let go of my dreams lost and exorbitant expectations. Once I looked honestly at my new normal, it opened the door to fresh possibilities.

What is can be painful but it's the birthplace for peace and love.

In the good times, I immersed myself in love. The love I felt for John and me, for my circumstances, for everyone around me, even for the stuff that still caused me physical and emotional pain. I know now that real love, with real compassion and forgiveness, is a second-to-none healer.

I now practice self-care. This puts wellness into my own hands. It's all about diet, exercise, letting go of toxic people and most importantly, spiritual meditation for myself and John and our planet. More and more, I'm letting go of the bad energy resulting in far fewer burdens and negative thoughts that make me sick. A gift to everyone, especially myself.

The greatest transformation for me is that I trust my gut and inner-wisdom to lead the way in my work, life and wellness. This is still a work in progress but the impact of trusting myself is so profound it makes each of my days richer. I am awash, once again, in beauty and appreciation.

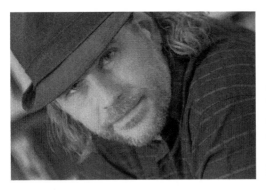

Dennis Maione
(Canada)
Wholeness and
advocacy

I'm an author, teacher, public speaker, healthcare and patient advocate and part-time church pastor with a passion for good health. More than that, I'm committed to helping people find personal wholeness despite their situations.

I came by my interest in patients, patient care and the quest for wholeness through my own journey from wellness to disease and back again. I have a genetic mutation called Lynch syndrome—a condition shared by 1.1 million people in North America. Lynch syndrome is greatly under-diagnosed. Only 5-10% of people with this mutation realize they have it. Unlike the genetics that make eyes blue or hair black, this mutation predisposes the carrier to an elevated risk of cancers in various organs. The rates of risk vary, depending on the Lynch type (there are at least five), the organ (highest in the colon and the uterus) and the individual with the mutation (their biochemistry and circumstances).

Having Lynch syndrome resulted in two colorectal cancers for me, the first in 1993 and the second in 2007. Both required surgery and both required self-advocacy to protect me from some of my doctors and from a healthcare system which seemed bent on drastically reducing my quality of life. I documented my over 20-year journey through cancer, self-education and struggle for personal wholeness in my book, What I Learned from Cancer (2014, PromptterstoLife.com).

I came to recognize the importance of advocacy for those who do not know they have this mutation and for those who are called previvors (those who have the mutation but have not yet had cancer), in large part through the experience of my own children. I was already a father of three when I first learned I had MSH2 Lynch syndrome and that each of my children had a 50% chance of having inherited this mutation. Given my own early onset of colorectal cancer, my wife Debra and I had each child genetically tested to ensure that measures could be taken to reduce the occurrence and minimize the effects of any cancer in our children who turned out to be carriers. I now advocate for my one child to whom I passed on this mutation.

Outside of advocacy, I write books, blogs and plays, speak to cancer patients, survivors and healthcare providers, teach memoir writing in high schools and generally try to keep out of trouble. For more information about projects in the works, my speaking schedule and how to get my books, check out my website at DennisMaione.com.

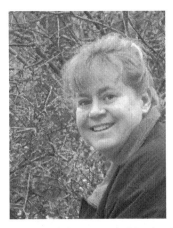

Elizabeth Gross (USA)
Life-ending? Not yet!

I'm a wife, Swiftie Mom, wildlife gardener, good news sharer, chocoholic, dream accomplisher and author of the award-winning book, Dream Accomplished: A Story of Cancer, A Mother's Love & Taylor Swift. Most days you can find me typing on my laptop or singing along to Taylor Swift songs with my husband and daughter as we garden on our 'Little Lot' in Northeast Ohio. I'm also a cancer-battler and invisible illness warrior.

I have a rare, chronic cancer called myeloproliferative neoplasm disorder essential thrombocytosis (ET for short). Before I get into that, let me tell you a bit about who I was 'before ET.' I am a graduate of The Ohio State University where I met and married my husband. I hold dual degrees in Greenhouse Management and Production, and Floral Design and Marketing. Through the years, I have held a multitude of jobs in the horticulture industry ranging from floral designer to botanical garden nursery manager, on to President of our family wildlife gardening design and installation company, "Lots of Life on a Little Lot." I love plants and wildlife and enjoy helping others learn about and love them all too.

In the fall of 2011, I noticed how fatigued I felt. I'd had a busy summer, juggling gardening clients and an active 7-year-old, and chalked it up to that. As the fall continued, I could not alleviate the fatigue and noticed other ailments cropping up as well. There were bruises, I had more intense migraines and I couldn't see well. My husband encouraged me to get a checkup and my family doctor thought I had depression. I disagreed and she reluctantly ran blood tests at my request. The labs came back with elevated platelets and low vitamin D. Not knowing what that meant and again, not really concerned, she scheduled me to see a blood doctor (hematologist) the following month. My husband and I felt that was too long and randomly chose a different hematologist from our network of insurance providers.

The next morning, I was diagnosed with symptoms of transient ischemic attack (warning stroke or TIA). I was rushed to the hospital to begin oral chemotherapy to lower my (blood clotting) platelet numbers, as my combined symptoms indicated a rare blood cancer that put me at high risk for clots, stroke and heart attack. In that instant, my life changed forever.

I remained in the hospital for 10 days, beginning my first real experience in dealing with doctors, unknowns, differing opinions, tests, surgeries, ultrasounds and bone marrow biopsies. Before this, my health, and my family's had been fine. The only time I'd been in the hospital was to have our daughter and my naïve thinking was still in place, "If you're sick, go to the doctor; they fix it and you get well." Now, I know better.

Over the next two years, I underwent every test under the sun and saw twenty-seven doctors across the United States including world-renowned heads of departments in neurology, cardiology, oncology and hematology. All but two agreed on my diagnosis and treatment plan.

I feel I've aged from 40 to 100 overnight and daily I slog through a litany of symptoms that seriously limit what I can do. We've had to adjust everything in our lives as my brain easily muddles and energy drains out of me like a deflating balloon. Frustrating? Yes. Scary? Yes. Life-ending? Not yet!

I hope that as you read this you can do as I've done and focus on that last thought, "Not yet!" Those words can lead you in the best direction of your life. They have for me! My journey has opened new windows of opportunity to help others, even with limitations, and I know somehow yours has too!

To find your path, think back. What was your first thought when you heard your diagnosis? What matters most to you in your life? Now hold onto those thoughts and combine them with the words – "Life-ending? Not yet!" That will give your life a direction on which to focus positively; it's what you still want to accomplish in your life.

My first thought after I heard, "You have cancer," was of our daughter. My focus and goal became making her dream to meet Taylor Swift come true and after much determination I was finally able to say, "Dream Accomplished!" I can't describe the enormity of that moment or feeling. It was like a match lit a fire in my soul. I knew in my heart that even in my darkest hour, I was still capable of anything. You are, too.

Read more of our story in my book, <u>Dream Accomplished: A Story of Cancer, A Mother's Love & Taylor Swift</u>, and visit me on my websites: dreamaccomplished.com and lotsoflifeonalittlelot.com.

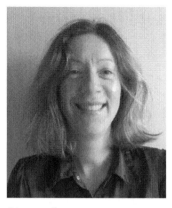

Elizabeth Turp (UK)
Denial is not helpful

I've been disabled by chronic illness half of my adult life. I had been active, healthy and enjoyed a career that I loved. Then at 31, after a very stressful year, I developed myalgic encephalomyelitis/chronic fatigue syndrome (ME/CFS). Five years later, an undiagnosed gynaecological problem I'd had since age 12 became severe.

I hadn't felt well for a while, but things got bad; I realised that I was holding onto door frames to stand up. Luckily, I was quickly diagnosed with ME/CFS. I did things to prevent deterioration and after a few years I was able to work part-time, relatively symptom-free by extreme pacing and living within a limited 'energy envelope.'

I began to suffer worsening pain and after twenty-four years of symptoms was diagnosed with endometriosis. I hemorrhaged during surgery to remove cysts, nearly dying on the operating table and was left in chronic pain. The fatigue became disabling again and after developing back pain, I was diagnosed with fibromyalgia. I've had to radically change how I live and work, coming close to losing everything several times.

I feel like I have a permanent flu. These conditions are complex and not well understood by doctors, so I've learned to self-manage. I experience limited mobility, nausea, brain fog, extreme fatigue, muscle weakness and disordered sleep. I'm unable to find words, have memory problems and am sensitive to noise and light. My conditions affect everything and going outside my stamina level, even a tiny bit, will increase symptoms. Living with these fluctuating, unpredictable symptoms made worse by everyday activities is extremely difficult.

I've made changes in my life to continue working as a counsellor while managing my symptoms. I've educated colleagues about my health, sought support from disability advocates and invoked Equality Law to implement 'reasonable adjustments' (changes to work practices, such as working in one place and having greater gaps between clients). Eventually self-employment became the best option.

I take a 'can do' stance and accept the difficult emotions that come with the restriction, uncertainty and isolation of long-term illness. As a mental health professional, I know suppressing darker feelings only makes life harder. I'm a huge advocate for honesty, answering the routine question from loved ones, "How are you?" with the truth. I offer clients with chronic illness and pain the acceptance, empathy and understanding that I have found so rare and precious on my own journey. I am counselling with the acknowledgement of the courage, resilience and skills they use to just exist.

Living with invisible illness comes with difficulties, both practical and emotional, and being heard and fully understood can be transformative. Denial is not helpful. I assist others in accepting their health issues, so they can develop self-management, assertiveness, pacing and stress reduction strategies. I give talks to patient groups, and train professionals on the impact of long-term illness on mental health and how to support people with chronic conditions.

I started writing about ME/CFS as a way of coping with the ignorance and hopelessness I encountered. A colleague heard about my writing and asked if I was interested in contributing to a series of books to help people understand complex health conditions. Chronic Fatigue Syndrome/ME: Support for Family & Friends was published in 2010. I was grateful for the opportunity to increase understanding about this condition and the 'difficult' topics: relationship problems, sex, suicide, guilt and shame.

It wasn't until my fibromyalgia diagnosis that I learned about the underlying neurological dysfunction in ME/CFS/fibromyalgia and am now hopeful about improving my quality of life. I use multiple strategies to cope: pacing, mindfulness meditation, nutrition, hormone treatments, exercise, sleep hygiene and physiotherapy. I've received shiatsu, counselling, acupuncture, massage and thoracic spine mobilization. I will always have pain but it doesn't rule me.

Life is completely different now and wonderful in ways. I maintain a good work-life balance with room for rest and enjoyable activities, better relationships and less stress. There has been a lot of loss along the way, of people who are unable to show care, of spontaneity, financial security, of certainty, the chance to have children, of freedom. Letting go of a conventional life doesn't mean you'll never achieve anything or have a life again. I've done more that I'm proud of as a sick person than I ever did while well, finding ways to do the right thing for myself and still have purpose. I've been working on my second book about living well with chronic illness for years. I think it will now have a different ending.

Visit my website, http://www.elizabethturp.co.uk, for further information about my work and articles on living well with chronic health problems and mental health.

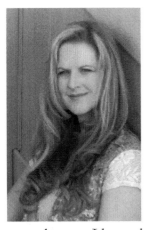

Erica Gayle Rogers (USA)
My disease empowers me

Currently living in rural west Texas, I am a mother of 7 beautiful children and wife to an amazing husband. I grew up on a farm in west Texas and have always enjoyed rural life. Although my later years have placed me in several states, I have always lived a simple, quiet life and have recently returned to my forever home. Motherhood and home life keep me busy but I am so lucky to have the continued support of my extended family as well as my husband and children.

I obtained a Bachelors in Education and MBA through Western Governor's University. I used to be energetic, rowdy and always on the go. I would jump at the chance to take on new challenges and met obstacles with a "can do" attitude.

My life changed when I received my diagnosis of relapsing-remitting MS in June 2015. My left eye had become blurry. Then one morning, I woke up and could not feel the left side of my chin, gum and cheek. I saw my optometrist who found my blood pressure was dangerously elevated; the doctor thought I was having a stroke and sent me to urgent care. A CT Scan was done and blood was drawn but all came back normal. Then an MRI of my brain was ordered and my doctor suggested that I see a neurologist.

At that time, I lived in a very rural part of northwestern Kansas. I found a neurologist in Denver, Colorado, 3½ hours away that could give me an appointment that week. The doctor found two lesions on my brain and suspected multiple sclerosis. However, diagnosis of MS could take some time. He ordered 5 days of IV steroids, an evoked potential test for my vision and an MRI of the cervical spine to check for additional lesions.

I went over the results of the tests with the doctor in July. Two lesions were found on the cervical spine and not only was there a significant delay of the optic nerve in my left eye but my right eye showed delay, too. A diagnosis of relapsing-remitting multiple sclerosis was confirmed and I had to start treatment immediately to delay the disease. I had to give myself injections 3 times a week...for the rest of my life. I was devastated but determined.

Since the day of diagnosis, I have lived by my motto that I will not let MS control me; it will EMPOWER me. I became inspired to create a plan for a non-profit organization to provide resources to MS patients that might not be available through traditional assistance programs. This work keeps me excited, positive and passionate about helping others.

I encourage every person facing adversity to discover how they can impact the lives of others. Find something that gives you joy and dive into it with your whole heart. Find comfort in those who love and care about you and do not get discouraged. Every effort makes a difference, big or small. I'm hoping that with continued diligence and passion, I can help many others like me.

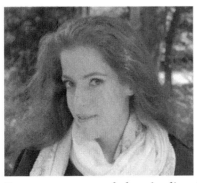

Grace Quantock (UK)
Anything is possible

At 18, I was far from home, from all I had known and lost in a foreign land.

It was strange and deeply disorienting. I didn't speak the language. I couldn't make myself understood. I didn't know how I'd ended up there; I had no power and couldn't see a way to get home. Every move seemed to be a faux pas that took me deeper from all I knew. I couldn't get it right and every day was wrong. I was objectified; people were more interested in my body than my feelings. I was discriminated against and judged. I was a second-class citizen in this new land and it hurt to be on the wrong side. It felt like every day I shed more of my identity. I was deeply scared. And there was the pain.

Let me explain. It had all started so innocuously; I was volunteering at a summer camp when I came down with something that felt like the flu. I was feverish, exhausted and after the sunny days on an animal sanctuary in Kent, England, it felt like perhaps I'd overdosed on sunlight.

In that moment, so full of light and youth, something shifted and I entered a new world, one of pain and internal awareness. Parts of me I'd never known began to hurt and it was the beginning of an intimate knowledge of my body and my own life. I had entered the "kingdom of the sick". *

It was a cold, grey February day when the doctor looked at me across the cluttered desk and told me the pain, fatigue, cognitive dysfunction and muscle weakness I was experiencing were permanent. But that's only part of the story. I was diagnosed with a long list of autoimmune conditions. Everything from my toe joints to my hypothalamus had struggles. My prognoses were dire. Because I wanted more. Because there is somewhere between desperately ill and miraculously cured: I'm living there, healing there, working and playing there...

The disabilities are just the footnotes; I am the adventure story. I decided to stop seeing myself as 'only' a sick chick, to hand back all the judgements and projections that society and the media heaped upon me. Instead of seeing my dreams crushed, beyond my grasp, I carved a new life, rising from the ashes of old dreams and blaze my own trail to new possibilities.

My joyous work emerged from my experience of illness: bed bound and hurting, letters became my link to the outside world. Until you are sick, imprisoned in your own home, in your own body, it is hard to understand how important mail is. I made Healing Boxes – gifts of information, support and healing goodies for friends and family. I couldn't find healing boxes in the UK; I continued to make my own and more and more people requested them. After a cancer scare at 22, I decided to stop being afraid and start living my dreams and so my entrepreneurial journey began.

Today, I am a trailblazing wellness coach; I write, teach and speak internationally on living well with pain, illness and life crisis. I'm the founder of Healing Boxes CIC and The Phoenix Fire Academy. A Future Young Leader of Wales Award recipient, Entrepreneur Wales Awards and Great British Entrepreneur Awards finalist and featured in The Hay Festival, Positive News, Gala Darling, TEDx, Huffington Post and The Times of London. I've been recognized as a trailblazer by thousands of people who have seen me speak and participated in my programs. I love what I'm doing and am so grateful to find such joy in my work.

The best advice I never had is to do it your way, not the 'right' way, because what works best for your body and life will be most successful for you. Look at what you love to do and how you work best. Working around your needs makes your work right for you. Blaze your own trail and do it your way. The one thing I did right was to reach out and ask for help. I didn't throw money at my business, I asked questions instead.

If you meet an amazing photographer, an online friend with an engaged social media following or someone with the qualification you dream of; reach out and ask them about it. Ask for a reading list and introductions to other people they recommend. Thank them and then act on the information you receive. Follow up on it all, then go back and (concisely) report your process and send a thank you card.

Step up and begin. Launch. It will never be perfect, you can refine as you grow but the world needs the revolution you have inside you right now.

* Susan Sontag, nybooks.com/articles/1978/01/26/illness-as-metaphor/

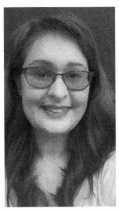

Jo Southall (UK)
Living creatively expands my identity

I'm an independent occupational therapist. This wasn't my original plan. I was always super sporty but at the age of 18 while working in the outdoor adventure industry my life changed drastically. After months of increasingly frequent joint injuries, constant increasing pain and horrendous fatigue, I was diagnosed with hypermobile Ehlers-Danlos syndrome (H-EDS). H-EDS is a genetic connective tissue disorder causing symptoms such as joint laxity, chronic pain and fatigue. In my case the joint laxity was extreme. I'd always been flexible but suddenly I couldn't control it. My joints dislocated frequently and often I found myself suddenly on the floor.

I struggled with a loss of identity for a long time after my diagnosis. While my body failed me the part of me that remained the same was my creativity. I had always loved arts and crafts and was usually surrounded by beads, cotton, glitter and glue. I started making jewelry, passing many a pain-filled hour with buttons and beads in my own little world.

I also started using my creative energy in managing my deteriorating health. I spent months learning obsessively all I could about H-EDS while trying to hold on to my 'old' self. Despite this, from the age of 19 on my health declined dramatically. I was a dancer, I did Parkour (the sport of negotiating obstacles by running, jumping and climbing) and taught rock climbing. By the age of 22 I had left my old job behind and pursued a degree as an occupational therapist, despite a few health set-backs.

I've been using a wheelchair part-time to manage my joint problems and fatigue and I've gradually learned to deal with all the new symptoms my body throws at me. I now have chronic fatigue, migraines, postural orthostatic tachycardia syndrome (POTS), heat intolerance and loads of food intolerances among other issues.

I have more control over my health and have stopped obsessing over the loss of the 'old' me. I focus on the 'new' me and what I CAN do as opposed to what I CAN'T. Don't get me wrong, I still miss the old me and I've lost more than a job! But the 'new' me is pretty cool, too.

Living creatively and problem-solving my way through life has allowed me to expand my identity. Along with my career in occupational therapy, I've been part of a wheelchair basketball team, I've taken up yoga and I run a successful blog where I teach self-management skills to people with chronic conditions. I've also volunteered for the Hypermobility Syndromes Association (HMSA), a charity that helped me through my darkest moments.

Finally, during one of the sporting accidents leading up to my diagnosis I found the courage to tell a special someone my feelings; after a few hours at the local hospital I realised he felt the same way. My partner, Addz, and I have been together ever since. Without the nasty H-EDS-related accident who knows if we would have gotten together? Who knows if any of this would have happened?

My creativity is still alive and kicking and I love it! My Facebook page, **The Creative Life of JBOT**, has allowed me to showcase my creative work and Etsy helps me shift my creations to loving new homes! Working on jewelry pieces for commission is a great way to step out of my comfort zone creatively. I manage to make jewelry even at my worst; it's something that will always hold a special place in my soul.

In the last few years I have turned my creative eye towards photography. Developing my photography and editing skills has not only given me many happy hours watching birds, bees and butterflies but I've stayed connected with the dance and parkour community, not as a participant but as photographer! Living life through a lens can have beautiful results.

Possibly my favourite creative venture has been nail art! I have a nail polish collection to rival most makeup counters. I even use my nails as a pacing tool for managing fatigue; if I notice my nails are a mess, I know I've been working too hard and resting too little!

Using social media has helped me share my experiences and learn from others. Consequently, one thing has really struck me; disability might close doors, but it also opens them. Some of the doors it opens are amazing! Learn about my career at www.jboccupationaltherapy.co.uk.

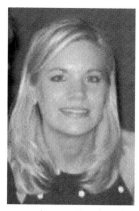

Kari Ulrich (USA)
Accept change

Before being diagnosed with a chronic illness, I worked as a supervisor in a multispecialty clinic, then as a registered nurse with both pediatric and adult emergency room experience. In April 2007, my life put on the brakes.

I was diagnosed with a rare vascular disease called fibromuscular dysplasia, as well as Ehlers-Danlos syndrome, a connective tissue disorder. What started out as exercise intolerance and a swooshing sound in my ear turned out to be something much more serious. I had symptoms for many years but nobody had really put it together until I was thoroughly evaluated at Mayo Clinic in Rochester, Minnesota. Through this journey, I learned that vascular disease in young women is under-diagnosed. I also learned that there was a great need for patient support and advocacy.

Looking back to my early twenties, I suspected that the symptoms I was experiencing were not something every young adult faced. I always looked healthy on the outside; I was judged by my appearance, not by the symptoms that I was describing to my health care provider. I had been diagnosed with hypertension at a young age but the cause wasn't investigated. I suffered from a multitude of connective tissue symptoms, as well as abdominal pain, but no one put the pieces of the puzzle together.

Almost two decades later at age thirty-nine, through a coordinated evaluation at Mayo Clinic, I finally found the answers to what had been causing my symptoms.

In July 2006, I started running and trained for a half marathon. I would run up to 10-13 miles. In the Spring of 2007, I felt short of breath going up stairs and could run only one mile. I developed palpitations and felt dizzy just sitting at my computer. I also had a loud swooshing in my ears. I saw a cardiologist for my frequent skipped heartbeats and he heard bruits (noisy pulses) in my carotid (neck/head), epigastric (upper abdomen), renal (kidney) and femoral (thigh) arteries.

I was diagnosed with a rare vascular disease called fibromuscular dysplasia (FMD) with brain aneurysms. My FMD affects several of my vascular beds. The arteries that supply my kidneys are affected causing high blood pressure. The arteries supplying my carotid arteries are also affected causing neck pain, headaches, dizziness and a loud swooshing sound in my ears. For most, FMD is an invisible illness which makes diagnosis even more of a challenge for physicians.

My abdominal pain was caused by the narrowing of my celiac artery from the FMD, as well as median arcuate ligament syndrome (MALS) which compresses that artery. For many years, I had symptoms of weight loss, nausea and food avoidance. At times, the pain was so severe that I would forgo eating meals with my family. Mayo Clinic took the time to put the pieces of the puzzle together. I underwent a catheter angiogram which confirmed my FMD and MALS was diagnosed. In August of 2009, I went through a celiac bypass and bovine patch to my hepatic artery for treatment of MALS. I had a revision of my celiac by-pass in 2015.

Over the years my quality of life has changed drastically. Learning to accept that you have a chronic illness is not done overnight; it is a process of accepting change. You mourn your previous self and learn to celebrate your new self. This is not something that can be managed on your own. It takes a team of physicians, psychologists, friends and family. What made me happy before my illness makes me melancholy today. Now I find great joy in my family and home. I have made my home my oasis, surrounding myself with what I love.

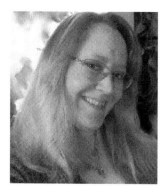

Katherine Dunn (Canada)
Find a way to enjoy life

I've lived with chronic pain since I was 10, constant pain since 2005. I have lumbar hernia, chronic sciatic pain, fibromyalgia and chronic fatigue syndrome.

I married and had my two children in my early twenties; a blessing, for those were my best years! We live in the Laurentian mountains of Quebec, Canada, with our giant Wooly Husky, Balto. I grew up with intimate knowledge of chronic illness: my mother has had lupus for over 40 years and my sister, my confidant and friend, has had migraine her entire life. I think this experience along with the built-in support group they provide has helped make me stronger and living easier.

I was a teacher and private tutor. I don't know what I will do in the future beyond my creative hobbies, but I'm working on a Master's in Education, focusing on Disability Services. I am passionate about the subject though research and writing are a challenge with fatigue, brain fog and pain.

There have been months when I was mostly bedridden. When my leg feels almost too heavy to move, I walk with a cane or a walker. I manage to go shopping in a mall or box store by using a wheelchair or mobility scooter. I also have a walker with a seat that converts to a transport chair. It's wider and more comfortable than most rollators and allows me to alternate between sitting and walking (as long as I have someone to push me). No matter the obstacles I face, I find a way to work with it.

Reading "The Spoon Theory" story on Christine Miserandino's website really hit home. It provided an easy way for me to express my level of pain and fatigue to others without bursting into tears. Online, I also connected with other people with chronic illness, known as "spoonies" and I joined support groups. The additional support makes a big difference in my quality of life!

My best tool for surviving chronic pain is my creativity, a true blessing. It helps me relax. Whenever I sketch, scrapbook, take photographs or make jewelry I am completely absorbed in the project and I forget my pain. I must be careful because I can sit for too long while creating, causing more pain. I choose supportive positions like lying in bed and set an alarm reminding me to get up and move. There are times when I crave a day off from monitoring my position but I remind myself of the progress I've made by honoring my limitations.

Instead of applying for standard disability, I applied for financial aid as a student with a major functional disability, which allowed me to receive loans as bursuries, equivalent to a grant. Disability Services has been a blessing with many extensions and services. That's why my thesis focuses on improving disability services for online universities; paying it forward. Contact me to find out more about getting a Canadian government grant to study for free (if you're permanently disabled). Balto_mama@icloud.com

I began making jewelry in 2010. I doubt I could have persevered without a creative outlet. I adore designing, creating and sharing. I work on my jewelry as often as I can! I love to see people smile when they see my creations.

As with most chronic illness warriors, I struggle financially. Every Christmas I focus on one creation for gifts, which helps. In 2018, a carpal tunnel injury flared badly. I couldn't make jewelry, but I reminded myself that I am the queen of accommodations! I found a way to make crystal snowflakes with my left hand! I also began to pain with watercolour. Holding the brush loosely, I was able to paint cards that were appreciated. I decorated my room with new creations, a reminder that no matter the obstacle, I will find a way to persevere and create.

Pain has taught me to find a way to enjoy life. Waiting for surgery or a cure will not help me fight depression today. I've become the queen of accommodation and set about building my best life day-by-day. I still have a way to go, but I am content. With my limitations, being content is amazing!

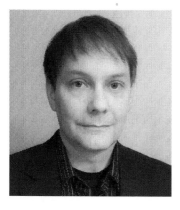

Ken McKim (USA)
One day at a time

I never thought I'd become an advocate for the chronically ill. I had worked at the Nevada Hospital Association doing IT support and helping administer the Health Resources and Services Administration Hospital Preparedness Grant. My wife, Corina, and I threw parties, went to roller derby matches, lived at the gym. At one point, we had a house. It was a very different life than what we have now.

I've suffered from manic depression for probably my entire life. I was hyperactive as a kid; at six I was medicated and doing biofeedback to help with depression and to calm me down enough to sleep. At ten, my mother died and I got into fist-fights at school. Not the best of times.

Some days my anxiety is still off the charts; the medication I'm on takes care of the worst of the depression and helps keeps me "even" but at times during the week, I feel like curling up into a ball and weeping. My insurance doesn't cover mental health care. My meds are free but seeing a psychologist or psychiatrist is not. I'm just winging it.

I began having cluster headaches in the early 2000's making work a challenge. I had a cluster headache every other day like clockwork and the day after I'd be lucky if I could work a full shift.

During that time, I was continually misdiagnosed with migraine. One of the nights my wife had to drive me to the ER, the on-call doctor recognized my symptoms as cluster headaches. Suddenly, all the pieces fit. Not long after that we started trying things like oxygen therapy and then a concoction we called "cluster coffee" which if drunk at the onset of an attack would greatly lessen (and occasionally stop) the pain.

In 2010, my clusters disappeared. I have no idea why but you can rest assured that I don't take that for granted. I still get horrible "ice-pick" headaches but I'll take them over clusters any day! It was good timing, too, because around that time my wife's health took a turn for the worse.

Corina's Crohn's disease started to manifest around 2007, though we had no idea what it was at the time; it took years to get that diagnosis. Corina is a humorous, gifted artist. Unfortunately, her ability to create has been impacted by the disease. Her energy level is very low and in addition to the inflammation of her bowel (she has just enough colon to prevent her from having an ostomy bag) her hands hurt almost to the point of tears. We've tried everything. One medication almost worked but showed signs of damaging her liver so it was discontinued.

I focus my energy on helping Corina manage her Crohn's. We're not as outgoing as we used to be; any kind of prolonged physical activity usually results in a gastrointestinal bleed for her. We watch a lot of television and when she feels halfway decent we do as much as we're able. She lost her job because of her illness (though the employers would never admit that) and we lost our house. Our health problems have changed our lives greatly.

The first video I ever produced, "The Slow Death of Compassion for the Chronically Ill", was a half-hour presentation I gave in my hometown of Reno, NV. It was based on my reaction to the reclassification/rescheduling of opioid-based pain medications from Schedule III to Schedule II, which I feel is one of the worst decisions ever made by the FDA and the DEA.

During the process of putting that talk together, I realized that my wife and I could not be the only people having problems explaining chronic illness to friends, family and co-workers. So began my "Don't Punish Pain" videos. I aimed to produce simple, educational videos that could be used as primers on various illnesses. I've made over fifty videos now with over 130K views on my channel which blows my mind.

I love creating videos. I think video is the best medium for conveying emotion, and if you do it well you can elicit an emotional reaction from the viewer. Emotion goes hand-in-hand with our capacity for empathy; if you want to motivate someone to action you've got to incite emotional investment in the topic. I think I'm good at that.

I have no idea what the future holds for us. I must take it one day at a time; sometimes one hour at a time. Maybe someone will see my work and be inspired to help develop it into a real show with a proper budget. I do this because of the amazing emails from people saying that through my videos they were finally able to help someone understand what they go through. Those emails give me hope. Maybe compassion can make a comeback after all. Maybe, just maybe, I can help the jaded cynics in society see that the chronically ill deserve the same shot at happiness and dignity as healthy people do. We'll see what happens.

View my videos at pajamadaze.com/blog/category/ken-mckim-feel-this-pain and on my YouTube channel - youtube.com/user/NVKen42.

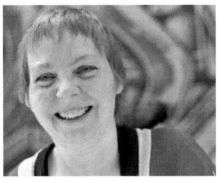

Lene Andersen (Canada) Being positive is a conscious choice

I don't remember a time before juvenile arthritis (JA). That is to say I have a handful of images that I can call up, moments from before I was four years old. This was when the first symptom of JA showed up. My left ankle swelled hugely so I couldn't walk. My parents thought it was from a particularly nasty mosquito bite. I remember my mother pushing me along a dirt road in a stroller while being aware that I was too old to travel that way.

I don't remember all the doctors who examined me over the next five years; who said there was nothing wrong with me and, in a novel twist, saying it was all in my mother's head. I don't remember the doctor who held my swollen hand in his and finally gave me a diagnosis when I was nine.

It's hard to sum up 50 years of living with chronic illness. Highlights include spending a lot of time in hospitals as a kid, almost dying from a JA systemic flare in my early teens and getting both hips replaced at 16. I had been stuck in hospital, lying in a bed for the previous two years. The surgery enabled me to sit again so I could go home with a power wheelchair and start living life. Another massive flare in 2004 brought me close to dying again but thankfully a new medication saved me. It was the first time in my life with this disease that an effective medication was available.

When I was a child my parents gave me a great gift by telling me I had a choice: I could laugh or I could cry. I knew instantly that I wanted to spend my life laughing. Putting this into practice is an ongoing journey. Having few memories of life before chronic illness and pain was probably helpful. This is my life; it is my normal. Wild flares aside, a certain middle range of pain and illness has always been the way things were.

I was born and raised in Denmark, moving to Canada with my family in the early 1980s. The Danes are a stoic people not prone to emotional outbursts and my family instinctively deflects into humor. Terrible jokes and gallows humor are a huge part of my coping arsenal. Following my big flare ten years ago this morphed into an acute awareness of joy and beauty. Having gazed into the abyss and seen the abyss looking back, flashing sharp teeth, and then escaping its bite, brought me a new and wonderful perspective on life.

In the last ten years I've created a much different life, in many ways becoming the person I always wanted to be. This has meant fulfilling my lifelong dream of being a writer and published author, as well as a photographer and chronic illness advocate. Most of all it means just plain enjoying life.

I have battled depression and sadness for much of my life because of chronic illness. Focusing on the positive has changed that, helping me to create a life filled with joy. Being positive isn't a mindless Pollyanna approach but a conscious choice (often several times a day). It has made it much easier to live with the curveballs chronic illness throws my way. It helps me to laugh. Every day.

You can find me online at my award-winning blog, The Seated View www.theseatedview.com as well as the website for my book <u>Your Life with Rheumatoid Arthritis: Tools for Treatment, Side Effects and Pain</u> www.yourlifewithRA.com. You can email me at lene@yourlifewithra.com.

Photo credit: Sofia Kinachtchouk

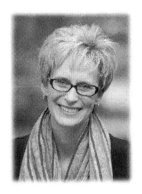

Louise Bibby (Australia)
Pursue passions and purpose

My journey with myalgic encephalomyelitis or chronic fatigue syndrome (ME/CFS) and electro-sensitivity has involved triumph and despair both psychologically and physically. I wouldn't be who I am today without having gone through it. I do acknowledge that it's been unfair and has destroyed parts of my life.

From the start, I've been driven to pursue my passions. I believe that a lost sense of purpose and identity impact people with chronic illness contributing to our grief. Part of my mission is to inspire others to follow their passions and regain or discover their purpose in life.

I was diagnosed with ME/CFS in 1992. I didn't believe it because I wasn't bed-bound. At times during those early years I seemed to recover, traveling with my future husband and working as a journalist. The full-time work lasted only four months though before I became so ill that at 22 I was forced to move back in with my parents.

I spent 2½ years recovering before starting a part-time Bachelor of Psychology degree (finishing in 3 years), then Honors full-time in 2000. The low contact hours helped but researching and writing a thesis (on the impact of ME/CFS on elite athletes' sense of identity) knocked my health around.

I wanted to be a psychologist but wasn't well enough to work part-time so I applied for and won a scholarship to do my Ph.D. in Psychology. I researched quality of life in people with ME/CFS which I could do in my own time.

In 2002, I was the healthiest I'd felt in years travelling with my husband to Disneyland, Calgary and the Caribbean. When we got back I became pregnant with my daughter. We hoped I'd be one of those people with ME/CFS who improved in pregnancy. Instead, I started experiencing severe headaches along with ear and face pain when I used my old laptop. This had been an issue with newer computers as well as mobile

54

phones but as the weeks rolled on everything electro-magnetic caused me pain - even the car!

I thought I was going crazy but I knew my nightmarish symptoms were real! My ME/CFS symptoms continued and with indigestion and 'morning' sickness, I couldn't lay down or lean back in a chair. Those 9 months and the 18 months that followed were my darkest period. Luckily having had training in counselling and suicide intervention I realized I needed help. I sought counselling which did help and took anti-depressants which didn't.

Unfortunately, it all took its toll on my husband; my soul mate, best friend and tower of strength through 12 years of illness. With tears, we separated. I re-married too quickly and separated from my second husband amicably.

At my sickest, I felt most of the avenues to pursue my passions were gone. I've realized that was just a context based in grief; I can still follow my passions, just in different ways. Courses at Landmark Education empowered me to recreate my life and do things I once thought impossible. I now use computers and watch TV; I choose to follow my passions using these even though I get severe headaches. I deal with constant pain by using sleep (with sleep aids), massage, yoga and hot baths.

In 2013, I pursued my passion and started a blog/website, www.GetUpAndGoGuru.com where I write about my experience with ME/CFS and electro-sensitivity and share how others can live powerfully with chronic illness. I've also launched TheWellnessQuest.net, a site that covers wellness-related topics from a holistic perspective.

I'm a chronically ill mother with limited energy and time. My daughter and I have an awesome relationship despite the restrictions of my illness; she often needs only small amounts of quality time to feel satisfied. I'm also a believer in the potential of building passive income online. Because of my experience I decided to publish an eBook, 15 Minute Power Plays With Your Kids: How To Be A Better Parent In 15 Minutes A Day. I also compiled a huge, free Resource Guide to support parents in implementing simple ways to spend quality time with kids and created a website based on the book. In December 2013 my eBook and website went 'live' and in August 2014 the book was launched on Amazon Kindle where it hit #1 in its category!

As I love connecting with people and making a difference in their lives, I have become a Transformational Coach/Life Transitions Coach for people with chronic illness and PTSD. I'm growing my Transformational Coaching business, online and off, while also working with a coaching colleague on an empowerment podcast called Just Breeze. I am creating coaching courses as extensions of the podcast and growing TheWellnessQuest.net site while compiling my best blogs into a book. Though pursuing my passions and purpose via the internet causes pain, I live life fully and build financial freedom while I work toward total health.

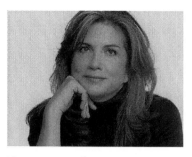

Martine Ehrenclou (USA)
Be a take-charge patient

I'm an award-winning author, patient advocate and speaker. My book, The Take-Charge Patient: How You Can Get The Best Medical Care, winner of ten book awards, empowers readers to become proactive and effective participants in their own health care. My mission is to bring to light the importance of being an advocate for oneself and others. Through my books, media interviews, published articles, blog, and lectures, I reveal insider information on how to interact effectively with medical professionals and navigate the health care system. I've interviewed over 200 physicians, nurses, other medical professionals and patients for my latest book.

Six months into my research for The Take-Charge Patient, I developed debilitating, chronic pain that lasted sixteen months and had to use every strategy in the book I was writing. I went from an advocate for others to an advocate for myself and became my own take-charge patient. After ten doctors failed to diagnose me correctly, my exhaustive research led me to the surgeon who finally diagnosed and cured me. I remain pain-free at the time of this writing.

I regularly publish articles on the topics of patient empowerment, patient advocacy, patient safety, successful communication in medical encounters, the collaborative relationship between patients and medical professionals, and other health/medical related issues. I am interviewed recurrently on national TV, radio, newspapers and magazines, including NBC News, ABC News, KCAL 9 News, NPR, Woman's Day, Family Circle, Los Angeles Times Magazine and many more. I also lecture at universities, hospitals, and health organizations, and write a blog.

I am also the author of the award-winning book, Critical Conditions: The Essential Hospital Guide To Get Your Loved One Out Alive.

Please visit my website, TheTakeChargePatient.com

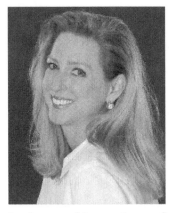

Mary Pettigrew (USA)
Passion and endless
possibilities

I am a late-blooming writer from Texas who specializes in poetry. I also have a background in music, performing arts and enjoyed 14 years as a special events planner in the private club industry. I graduated in 1990 from The University of North Texas starting off as a music major (voice) but I wasn't "feeling" it. I changed direction and happily ended up graduating with a B.S. in Hotel/Restaurant Management. I was healthy, eventually married, a stepmother of two and had a fun, successful career in the food and beverage industry until 2001. Life as I knew it changed dramatically when I was diagnosed with multiple sclerosis.

I can't describe how lost I felt in those first years after diagnosis. I attempted to work a few more years but nothing connected quite right anymore so I was soon forced to quit. This disease affects everyone differently. I went through numb/tingly issues with my mobility intact but I was, and continue to be, an "invisible symptom" case. My MS enjoys messing with my brain. Anxiety, memory, mood changes, heat sensitivity and fatigue are debilitating and a battle ensues, especially when stressed. There has been some noticeable progression in my symptoms and I've had to switch medications many times. This can be quite fearful but common.

A few denial years went by as I dealt with this vile invasion by my "internal roommate." My husband couldn't handle my health changes; he hated every part of it and I don't really blame him. He avoided being around me when I was down. Sometimes I imagined I could hear him say, "I didn't sign on for this," "I can't understand any of it" and "She sure doesn't look sick." Eventually divorce and other challenges came into play. Those were rough days...rough years.

Looking back now, I know that I was suffering a nervous breakdown. Not yet had I thought to seek a professional therapist to help me purge

58

the noisy voices and conversations from inside my head. I began to write. I wrote little songs and played piano again. I taught myself acoustic guitar and it felt good, soothing. I had found a new form of therapy which enabled me to breathe again; a healing that didn't require a prescription. Re-invention of myself seemed plausible through these creative outlets. Music, reading and writing (primarily poetry) filled me with passion and endless possibilities. In fact, I've since begun to view my MS as a gift which forced me to focus on the important things in life; to find my sense of humor, ignite my passion and live.

I constructed a blog site for my creative writing musettemary.wordpress.com. I've had two of my poems accepted in the UK for inclusion in two books of poetry compilations, The Summer of Sport: Forward Poetry 2012 and Poetry Rivals Collection 2013. My disability-themed poetry has been published on various blogs and websites, including www.pajamadaze.com and www.disabled-world.com. I was interviewed, as well, for an article about art/creativity therapy and MS, for the National Multiple Sclerosis Society's Momentum Magazine (Summer issue 2013)!

In the summer of 2014, I created MSpals, a community for MSers completely administrated by MSers. I recruited others to help run various facets of MSpals and our organization has grown bigger and faster than I ever could have imagined. Besides the various social media connections we are involved in, we have been interviewed and included in Momentum Magazine. Our website mspals.org is also up and running! For those of us who can no longer work, this has given us inspiration, a sense of purpose in providing support for others and an important VOICE in spreading awareness about MS.

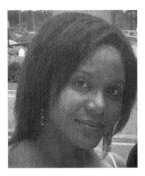

Melanie Styles (USA)
Inspired to inspire

My journey through chronic illness has been a long one, starting around age 5 with severe stomach aches and nose bleeds. I had swollen joints, irritable bowel syndrome with constipation, dizziness, even a large benign tumor in a salivary gland and another in my wrist. I remember getting migraine as a child. As a teen, I was told I had endometriosis and that I'd have difficulty getting pregnant. I had my first colonoscopy at 21. I've now tallied twenty official diagnoses and five surgeries.

I am ambidextrous and was identified as highly intelligent at an early age. Despite my health issues, I enjoyed activities including cheering, ballet, debate team and competing on a national level as a mock trial lawyer in high school and college. I graduated high school early in a time when it was discouraged and attended the University of Missouri. I was officially diagnosed with migraines while in college; those and other illnesses made it difficult to attend class. I married my high school sweetheart after my freshman year and despite having three children and illness, earned degrees in Spanish, Theatre and Dance, and Business. I worked in business for a few years after graduating then enrolled in graduate school.

My life's dream was to be a lawyer. I had trained and rubbed elbows with top lawyers and judges since my freshman year in high school. After having my fourth child, I saw that my passion wasn't for winning an argument; it was working with and helping people. I earned a Master's Degree in Education and loved working in education for ten years.

My doctor offered no real resolution to my laundry list of symptoms. Fibromyalgia was not a diagnosis option at that time. The holistic physician, however, offered answers that were widely unavailable in the United States. She prescribed a plan for detoxification, dietary changes and supplements that kept my fibromyalgia at bay for years.

I had a few migraines a month for about twenty years and then "my wheels fell off." I was hit on the driver's side door of my car at low speed. This accident completely changed the way my body experienced pain. Within a year, I had a hysterectomy.

Around that time, I also developed a seizure disorder called palatal myoclonus (PM); my brain tells the soft tissue separating my nose and mouth to vibrate. It's so violent that it causes the bones in my ears to vibrate, making me dizzy. The vibration is loud enough for others to hear. Many people report developing this condition after dental surgery. I've had extensive dental surgery; however, brain damage also showed up on a scan. The doctors thought the damage was due to the migraines. I thought it could be from extended oxygen deprivation as a test revealed decreased lung efficiency. Another theory was that the disorder could be related to the four concussions I've had.

I suddenly developed chronic daily migraine with severe sensitivity to light. I now required blackout curtains in my home, layered one upon another with regular curtains on top. I refer to my bedroom as "My Cave."

I feel that I am still very much in the thick of it. I am torn between the sadness and stress of not being heard or helped by doctors and the joy in my soul because I am alive. My family has accompanied me through every important journey and adventure. We continue to giggle and laugh our way through the most painful experiences. We get enjoyment out of making everyday life into a situation comedy and our favorite kinds of people are those who will play along.

I was lying in bed one night and felt inspired to start "Spoonie Style Guide," my video series for the chronically ill on YouTube. As I rarely leave my house and can barely talk on the phone now my major contact with others is through social media. I started my YouTube channel to inspire people with chronic illness to live, optimize their energy, have fun and do it in style!

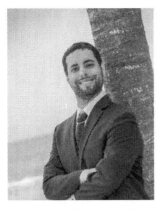

Michael Fernandez (USA)
Winning one battle at a time

For close to a decade, I was told everything from, "It's all anxiety" to "There's nothing more we can do, Mr. Fernandez, it's a matter of hours to days." I suffer from a plethora of tangled diagnoses. They range from cluster headaches, one of the most painful diseases known to doctors, all the way to Stage 3 EGPA vasculitis, formerly known as CSS or Churg-Strauss syndrome. I battle every day.

From the day I was born, the hospital has been a familiar place. My tiny body would not digest proteins properly. An allergy to a sulfa drug almost killed me, leaving me looking like a burn victim. By the age of eleven I had had seven surgeries to keep me from going deaf.

My hearing issues kept me from learning to read and write properly until second grade. Lacking sufficient support from the school, I taught myself to read Moby Dick.

At the age of 14, I became bedridden for three months with Epstein-Barr virus (mononucleosis). Somehow, I finished my Sophomore year of high school with high grades and my creativity and writing skills progressed. That summer with my first job, I struggled with fatigue. My regular headaches turned into cluster headaches that weren't diagnosed until 2014.

I was very close to graduation in college when things came to a screeching halt. Blood began to appear as I urinated or vomited following my workouts. Though I had bulked up through three years of body building, my hulking little brother had to carry me out of my dorm and take me home.

It took more than 40 unsuccessful medications and five specialists before we found someone capable of providing the care I needed. One look at my swollen extremities by one specialist led me to a highly-recognized rheumatologist who specialized in vasculitis.

I was diagnosed with an extremely rare and incurable disease called Churg-Strauss syndrome. At stage 2, I began treatment but it failed to stop the progression of the disease.

The fire in my belly is my desire to advocate not only for myself but for all who have chronic illness. If my story, my advocacy, my social media or website helps even one suffering person, all the hours of painful struggle are worth the effort to do it! The people with whom I connect - patients, caregivers, writers, artists and compassionate friends/family - keep my advocacy and life fueled.

I am grateful to Cam Auxer and her website pajamadaze.com, my wife Venus Hercules-Fernandez and my family for making my life as comfortable as it has been! I am also grateful to have a business that I love, Gold Glove Collectibles, selling sports memorabilia!

I write poetry when the pain is at its worst. To all who share my fight with pain - the true warriors winning this war one battle at a time - I dedicate this poem:

Dedicated to patients worldwide and Cam:

Chronic pain runs through my veins
Cold and damp it sometimes reigns
My thoughts my body feels so decayed
I might need to read my pain away
And let it all float away!
For, my friends, we flourish with talent
Hidden behind our pain is great intelligence
In the toughest of environments, we flourish
So, my friends, take it from me
Today all we need is a good read
Perhaps a blanket and some iced tea
Get comfy and read some comforting poetry.

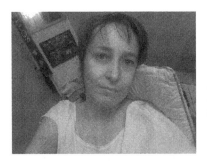

Miranda Brewster (UK)
The desire to create is strong

I've always had a need to create. As a child, I loved making things and found real satisfaction in producing a piece of artwork. As an adult I'm even more so and since I've come down with chronic illness and use the internet to access the world, I've discovered even more crafts to try.

In my twenties before I fell ill, I painted pots and made jewelry, selling pieces at local craft fayres along with some of my paintings. A friend put my miniature paintings in her shop and another friend invited me to her flower arranging parties to sell my creations alongside her arrangements.

I worked with children, running an after-school club, being a nanny and assisting at a dyslexia school, which gave me an opportunity to share my artistic skills and create wall displays for the school.

I had discovered my love of beading by this time. I was enchanted by the beautiful colours, shapes and the feel of them running through my fingers. I even loved the sound they made. Through books I taught myself stitches and techniques, and beading became my main hobby.

I had had bouts of bad health with no diagnosis nor reason. At 28, I developed pneumonia. My immunity had always been a bit weak. Common viruses would knock me down severely and I was frequently catching something but didn't think much of it. A second bout of pneumonia a year later, on top of a jaw infection and a minor head injury, caused a major health collapse. I didn't recover and was eventually diagnosed with myalgic encephalomyelitis (ME).

The level of exhaustion is beyond belief. I didn't know it was possible for the human body to feel so ill or be in that much pain without dying. It's called the "living death disease" and it totally claimed my life. I gave up work and moved in with my parents. For a long time I spent my days in bed, occasionally watching TV, unable to do much else.

Over a period of a year I improved enough to spend some time out of bed and use a computer. I taught myself touch typing, basic computer skills and soon became an inhabitant of the internet world.

It was there that I met Nigel in an online ME support group. Having both of us suffering from ME was challenging but we eventually managed to fly up and down the country to be with each other, and in 2005 we were married in a small, joyful ceremony.

I moved to the North East of England and my new life began. I wasn't well enough to work but was able to pursue my craftiness, adding glass painting and bead-making to my interests. My bead jewelry was even featured in a magazine!

We made the mistake of trying to live around our illness. I was forever pushing myself and kept having mini-crashes. My health deteriorated; in August 2010 I became bedridden.

Nigel's mum had early onset Alzheimer's disease which caused a huge amount of stress and sadness; four months after I became bedridden Nigel's mum died. I was heartbroken that I wasn't well enough to go to the funeral. Our life had become pure sorrow. For a year and a half, we desperately tried to survive but as I was refused professional in-home caregivers, we both deteriorated. When I was finally awarded that professional help, we had to share our home with people we didn't want there but desperately needed.

I continued to pursue my love of creating. Knitting and crochet was far more interesting than I had originally thought, previously passing them off as time-consuming and old-fashioned. On the days I was well enough they were ideal pass-times in bed and I wasn't losing beads in the sheets!

In 2011, my health took another dive. Crafts requiring a level of movement had to stop. Whereas I had been able to go downstairs once a day before, I haven't been downstairs since.

As part of coming to terms with our situation we created a website about ME using Nigel's web design skills. DozyDayz.co.uk was born as was my You Tube channel to make short videos about my experience and to share tips on coping with chronic illness.

Through social media and support groups we discovered wonderful people who have become valued friends. So many brave warriors all fighting to overcome limitations whilst supporting and encouraging one another! There is huge strength in weak bodies.

I began to improve for awhile so I continued with my drawing and became addicted to cross-stitch. Nail art captivated me, as well, so I bought tools and learned the techniques. I took up sketching mini portraits. Inspired by the exceptional instrumental skills of the 2CELLOS, music accompanied all the craft work I did. I would love to play the piano again and take up cello if ever I am well enough. Music, like art, is all about creating.

In 2014, I crashed again, this time severely. I suffered paralysis and stayed in hospital, too weak to swallow. All activity stopped and the years that followed became the worst days of my life.

I spent my days in a dark room with an eye mask against the light, earplugs against noise. For a while I couldn't speak, I couldn't lift my head off the pillow and, with great effort, could only just about roll onto my side. My ME had been bad before, but this was a totally new level. I was in a state of disbelief that I could feel so horrendously ill. I longed to escape the sheer terror and onslaught of symptoms and, at one point, begged Nigel to kill me, being unable to do it myself.

I didn't really want to die; I wanted to get better but I didn't think it was possible. It went on like that for years. The horror of those days haunts me. Though I have improved, I know I could go back there in an instant.

I have made progress with wonderful help from the amazing Thora Rain, a recovered ME sufferer. Although I'm still totally bedridden and must be spoon-fed, I am now able to sit up. I'm slowly, precariously crawling back to health and I weaken easily. With my current level of illness, I am unable to create; the cognitive function required is beyond me, holding a pen or pencil is difficult and repetitive movement causes pain and weakness.

The frustration is huge yet the drive to create is stronger than ever; I'm desperate to make things again. I try to satisfy this need by collecting pictures of crafts in a digital frame at my bedside. I'm inspired by others' talent. This feeds my motivation and enthusiasm and helps keep my interest alive. Nigel hangs cross-stitch kits where I can see them and I have a box of my beaded jewelry within reach.

I hope to soon get well enough to enjoy magazines and books again as well as watching tutorials on YouTube and the craft channel on TV. I want to do zentangle art and pencil carving, pin weaving, fibre art and yarn bombing. Button art, steampunk and upcycling. I want to learn seamstress skills, tatting, lace making, thread painting, soutache and shibori art... my interest is never ending. I have begun to draw small coloured circles, a few every now and then. It's lovely to produce colourful shapes again after being unable to for so long.

Taking up mindfulness as part of coping with my illness has made me realise that any project I undertake is about the process, not the result. I know now that I need not speed through to finish it, but instead take my time, be totally absorbed and savour every moment of creating. I believe my work will be better for it.

My priority is recovery and I can use my craft to help; artistic hobbies have proven benefits by triggering the body's relaxation response and boosting the chemicals of well-being in the brain. I shall continue to draw circles, I shall watch others create, I shall discover new ways of doing things and gradually, I will strengthen my ability and again become someone who creates.

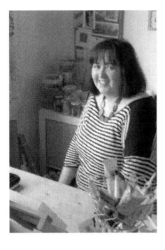

Nathalie Sheridan (UK)
Tomorrow is another day

Life was good. We had gotten married in Rome on a beautiful day in May 2009. We had plans to start a family and buy a house. By September that year we were in our perfect home located right near our friends.

Just three weeks later, the world began crashing down. A simple accident on the steps broke my ankle. No one was around and I lay out in the cold for an hour in agony waiting for an ambulance. By early the next morning I went home from the hospital on crutches. The only way I could climb the stairs to our house was not very dainty: I hauled myself up the stairs on my rear-end!

Weeks later the x-ray showed that the breaks had healed but my pain was still intense, the area swollen and an unhealthy colour. I had to get regular checkups and began physical therapy in January.

Eight months later my foot and ankle could still bear no weight. I noticed other changes in my health including memory loss, disorientation, over-sensitivity of the skin, chronic insomnia, depression, pins and needles, muscle spasms and constant pain with either freezing cold or searing heat sensations that travelled through to my bones. Opiate medication did nothing to stop the pain.

In September 2010, my orthopaedic consultant suggested that I could have chronic pain condition called complex regional pain syndrome or eeflex sympathetic dystrophy. Nerve blocks two months later were useless, just briefly relieving the pain. I tried every treatment available including physiotherapy, acupuncture, ultrasound, exercise and hot/cold therapy but none were successful in giving me relief.

Two years later, I discovered an in-patient pain management course at a neuro-rehabilitation hospital in London. Spending three weeks with other patients who knew what it was like to live with such pain was an incredible relief for me. Finally someone understood what I was going through! We were introduced to methods of physiotherapy, psychological therapy and relaxation/mindfulness training. From there I continued my care at a well-respected neurology hospital in Liverpool, The Walton Centre, one of the few UK hospitals that specialise in CRPS/RSD. Though different combinations of medicines, physiotherapy, desensitisation and mirror therapy were given to me, none relieved the pain. I am hoping a clinical trial may offer what I need.

I used to work as a Director's Personal Assistant in Central London. But now my cognition is that of an old woman. Working in a traditional job is out of the question. I am thankful for my smartphone that lets me create "sticky notes" and alarm reminders so I can keep track of what I need to do.

My passion is art – creating it in my studio and enjoying what others have created, visiting galleries and museums with my husband. There had been some interest in my paintings from family and friends. In the wee hours when I couldn't sleep, I researched the idea of selling my work and a few people had already commissioned a few pieces. I decided to go for it. My husband turned our spare bedroom into my art studio/library/office. I printed up business cards and put up a website, and in 2013, I started my own business: Nathalie Sheridan Arts.

I was diagnosed with an additional five chronic illnesses and had to juggle my art and life around flares and severe fatigue. Producing my artwork and keeping up with the website was difficult. I still try to handle much of my household chores and administration with the help of a cleaning person, but I finally had to make the choice to maintain balance over being successful. I made the tough decision to close my business in 2017.

Personal time and recreational activities with my husband are part of my striving for balance. We don't get to spend much time together because of his job so creating space for "us time" is a priority. We enjoyed a four-day vacation in Bath, a World Heritage site in South West England, which is full of architectural treasures and home to Jane Austen. Though in pain, I soldiered through so I could enjoy that quality time with him. We are making memories to last us through our golden years; chronic pain can't take that away from us.

I am also very grateful for the companionship of my rescued Jack Russell, Lucas. He is my baby, my Guardian Angel watching over me.

The mantra that keeps things in perspective for me is "Tomorrow Is Another Day." When depression, anxiety or pain make life tough, I draw a line through the day in my mental calendar and hope for a better tomorrow.

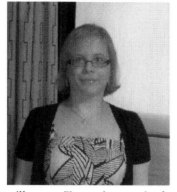

Rhiann Johns (UK)
Never give up your hopes and dreams

I cannot remember life before chronic illness. I've always had challenges and struggles because of the neurological condition with which I was eventually diagnosed. The pain and weakness in my legs was thought to be growing pains and I was too young to describe the dizziness and vertigo. Living with symptoms was my life. I battled through my childhood and adolescence and even earned a degree in Psychology despite the hardships that the symptoms created.

After graduating university, the symptoms began to worsen and the occasional bouts of dizziness and vertigo eventually became constant. The pain and weakness gradually intensified to the point where my legs regularly collapsed from under me. The weakness and pain as well as the balance problems became so severe that I had to use a walking stick. When I needed more stability, I traded the stick for a crutch. Nowadays, I often need a wheelchair when going out for long periods.

I was referred to and seen by a stream of specialists; from ENT to ophthalmology to neurology. I underwent numerous tests including an MRI to determine the cause of the symptoms. I was diagnosed with a long-standing brain stem lesion, in other words, scars on the brain stem probably from birth. After the diagnosis, I felt relief to finally explain my struggles since childhood and have validation that the symptoms weren't 'all in my head' as some doctors had concluded.

The diagnosis was vague and thus there was a distinct lack of information on how to treat the symptoms. The prescribed medication did little to dampen the pain and trembling in my legs or the dizziness.

Perhaps the most difficult aspect of living with a vague diagnosis was the lack of support. Search "long-standing brain stem lesion" and you'll find no information on the long-term prognosis nor where to connect with others living with a similar condition. The lack of social support compounded the loneliness and isolation I already felt from living with a long-term health condition. Due to the severity of the symptoms and the unpredictability of the weakness in my legs, I was unable to get out of the house on my own. It felt as if the condition robbed me of everything; my career prospects, my social life and finally, my independence.

I turned to the internet and joined the world of social media, searching for online support groups that could relate to my unique diagnosis. To my surprise, the chronic illness community was inclusive. Our situations and experiences of living with chronic illness were similar regardless of differing diagnoses. Gradually, I found a voice on social media describing my experiences and daily life with a neurological condition. Then someone suggested setting up my own blog where I could explore in further detail my neurological condition, as well as issues surrounding life with chronic illness and disability. I've always had a passion for writing but I wasn't sure that I could write my story in an eloquent fashion nor if anyone would be interested in reading it.

Slowly I gained a small but loyal following and the more people began to share links to my writing the more attention I gained within the chronic illness community. People left messages on the blog thanking me for putting their own feelings and experiences into words they could not express. I even received emails from people with brain lesions with whom I now keep in regular contact. My writing appeared in several magazines including The Pillow Fort Magazine, a digital publication for "spoonies" (people with chronic illness, fatigue or pain).

The blog and writing have been blessings in my life; for example, I now have a voice and purpose which I feared I had lost after my diagnosis. I'm now able to make friends with like-minded people who offer helpful, supportive words on a bad day. Through blogging and social media, I have found a place where I do not feel lonely or isolated.

If you are newly-diagnosed, don't believe that you are no longer able to do what you love. You may not be able to do things in the same way but with a little creativity you may find new ways of achieving goals. When the symptoms worsened, I thought I would never be able to travel again; waiting at an airport, then a flight, just felt like too much to handle. My parents and I decided to try cruising instead; now I've been on my third cruise, visiting Norway! Never give up your hope or dreams!

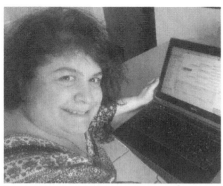

Sharon Yampell
(USA)
Make yourself your
priority

I was an executive secretary for companies around central New Jersey for the greater part of 26 years, interrupted by pregnancy, temporary disability and unemployment. This wasn't the work I studied for; I wanted to be a sports publicist. During my last year in college, I had a head-on collision that left me in chronic pain, changing the course of my life. It was nearly a year before I could look for employment and the first job that came along was assistant to a national accounts manager. One secretarial position led to another and another; I never became a publicist.

I was married to my first husband and my son was almost five when I was diagnosed with chronic Epstein-Barr virus (chronic fatigue syndrome) in 1995. Two years later I was diagnosed with fibromyalgia. I was on short term disability several times during those years then worked on and off for 19 years even after diagnoses of asthma and osteoarthritis. It wasn't until January of 2006 that I had to quit working as my health continued to deteriorate.

That August, my doctor pointed out that my bloodwork results showed that I had been sick with mononucleosis that spring, started getting better, then got it again before recuperating from the first case. I am one of the 12% of all chronic fatigue patients who has chronic Epstein Barr virus, also known as chronic or recurring mononucleosis. Eight years later, I was diagnosed with rheumatoid arthritis.

It was a major head-game to realize that I could no longer work at 40. I can't drive more than a half an hour and I miss day-to-day personal contact and having structure to my day (what I miss most). For over a decade now, a common cold becomes a long-term illness. At times, I've listened to my brain instead of my body and ended up in more pain, in bed for at least a week. I never know from day to day how I'll feel. My brain says go, but my body says no. I have learned to live my life written in pencil; I can't make definitive plans. The healthy world doesn't understand this. I miss the old me. I miss independence. I miss working.

Because of chronic pain, my sleep patterns are erratic; sometimes I require at least 1 or 2 long naps a day. Just to get any sleep at all, I used to rely on heavy pain medication and muscle relaxers that didn't always work. My pain levels made me a better forecaster of weather than the meteorologist, feeling a front come through 24-36 hours before it hits; I'm hardly ever wrong.

I still live with constant pain but rarely take medications unless the pain is beyond the scope of my normalcy. Pain is inevitable, suffering is optional! I know there's always someone who has it worse than I. Keeping that perspective gets me through my day.

I'm a completely different version of myself now and though my world got smaller, in some regards, I've learned to make myself my priority mastering the word "NO." It took two years to accept that my life has changed permanently; after that I learned to love myself as I am. That is a major victory. The other huge victory was accepting that it's okay to ask for help. Best of all, connecting through social media with others who have chronic illness has expanded my world!

As a child I was interested in genealogy as my grandparents were all children of immigrants. In 2005, I resurrected that interest and seriously explored my family tree. I wanted to know more about the family who left and/or stayed in Europe. Jewish records are difficult to find because Jews were exiled out of many countries during the war and family records were destroyed. I found an early version of Family Tree Maker and got started. I first viewed genealogical work as an exercise to keep my brain active. As time went on, it became a true passion; a high-tech scavenger hunt!

I reached the 2500 name count on my own tree and realized I could help others with their lineage. I joined numerous genealogy sites and called myself GenealogicalGenie charging by the number of names I discovered for others' family trees. My motto: "I am the GenealogicalGenie, I make your family history dreams come true."

What I'd like to tell people who are newly diagnosed or having a struggle with chronic illness is: Don't give up! There's always tomorrow. Don't be afraid to question what doctors tell you. Arm yourself with information to discuss possible alternatives for diagnosis and treatment. By doing this, you teach your doctor how you expect to be treated as a patient. You want your doctor to work with you, not for you, to coordinate your care. You must become your own best advocate.

I'm still the same compassionate, loving person I've always been but I'm more guarded now. I don't want pity; I want understanding. That's what everyone with chronic illness wants. We need to be a voice for each other.

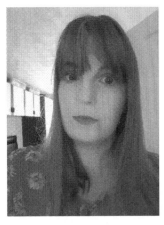

Siân Wootton (UK)
Find the silver linings

I'm Siân, an over-prepared enthusiast for organization and a lover of theatre. I certainly wasn't prepared when I was struck down with a chronic illness called myalgic encephalomyelitis. How can you be? It's not something you expect when in the prime of life.

I was one week away from finishing drama school, excited to be going on tour as an assistant stage manager when my body decided to give up entirely. I did not have the energy to even open my eyes or communicate for three days. I felt completely locked inside my body and very frightened. What was happening to me? Waking up in hospital after being tested for conditions such as meningitis, I was told I was suffering exhaustion and burn-out and that I needed to rest to help my body recover.

Four months went by and I was still feeling exhausted; everything seemed like a massive effort, physically and mentally. I'd gone from shifting heavy sets and retaining lots of information to feeling like the steel deck that I had been lugging around had fallen on me and I struggled to find the simplest word. Onlookers probably thought I was drunk as people tried to prop me up whilst I staggered about and fell asleep just about anywhere. Eventually, I was diagnosed with myalgic encephalomyelitis (ME).

It was good to finally have a diagnosis and know that life had not been ripped apart by my own error. At the same time, it was hard to accept that there was little that could be done and I might never get better. This became even harder when my health further declined and I was diagnosed with fibromyalgia, too. The house began to fill with all kinds of aids, my reliance on Mum's care increased and for me to leave the house I needed to use a wheelchair.

Spending most of my time inside the four walls of my bedroom was incredibly isolating. I needed to interact with the outside world and find others like me to help my mental health, before it took a downward spiral. I'd heard about support groups and had attended an ME clinic, but you must be physically able to get there. That is how the idea for my blog howtodealwithme.blogspot.com, came about. I wanted to write cathartically about my experiences whilst reaching out to other sufferers or family and friends of sufferers. I couldn't be the only one going through this! By sharing my blog through social media I've come to realise just how big the chronic illness online community is. There are thousands of people trying to make sense of their illnesses and looking for others who simply understand.

People in this community continually amaze me with their strength and positivity. They've helped influence the way in which I cope with this illness and remind me that, although our lives are by no means easy there is still plenty to laugh and smile about; an ethos I try to live by and convey in my blog posts. I now see my wheelchair as an enabler so I can spend a few hours during better days out of the house doing something fun or "normal" which simply wouldn't happen without it. Thanks to friends and websites like pajamadaze.com, I've taken up hobbies I can do in bed such as jewelry-making and scrapbooking. Learning a new skill and getting to see something I've created makes me feel like I can still achieve something. As someone that thought I'd never accomplish anything new after getting ill, that is a big deal. It's also fun making something nice for myself, my friends and my family.

I'm lucky enough to have travelled a few times since becoming ill which has helped bolster my belief that I can have a meaningful life. There had been times when just contemplating travel seemed impossible. That's why I encourage others through my blog (and this book) by sharing experiences, tips and advice about holidaying with chronic illness.

To me, life is still worth living. I try to remember that I remain the person I was, only my circumstances have changed. As I face different challenges, I try my best to live by the quote, "Every day might not be good but there is something good in every day." There's still plenty to be grateful for. Sometimes you must look a bit harder but there are still silver linings.

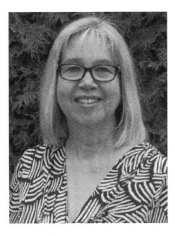

Suzanne Robins (Canada) Transform tragedy into triumph

I was in my early thirties when I began to experience health problems that would eventually be diagnosed as multiple sclerosis (MS) - a progressive neurological disorder that damages the central nervous system. I was a busy stay-at-home mom at the time with a thriving freelance writing business.

For me, insomnia was the first sign of trouble. I couldn't fall asleep or stay asleep - even when I was exhausted - and I was getting up countless times in the night with an urgent need to pee. Both issues are symptoms of MS but they weren't pieced together at the time. My doctor believed my bladder problems were caused by childbirth and encouraged me to do Kegel exercises to strengthen my pelvic floor. I thought my sleep was just being disrupted by my kids who were babies then and poor sleepers too.

Soon I was barely sleeping at all, so I was chronically fatigued and irritable. As it became more difficult for me to perform my duties as a mother and a freelance writer, I grew increasingly anxious. I started having panic attacks that would strike me out of the blue and take my breath away. Eventually, they became so frequent and severe that I had to be hospitalized. I spent three weeks on a psychiatric ward. I was diagnosed with clinical depression, put on an antidepressant and released to the care of a psychiatrist.

My symptoms gradually stabilized except for my bladder which continued to do its hyperactive thing. Everything was fine for several years, until I suddenly started having problems again - headaches, bouts of uncontrollable crying, acute sleep disruption and more panic attacks. The onset was so dramatic - and so inexplicable - that my psychiatrist thought there was something wrong with my medication. I had just filled a new prescription and he actually returned it to the manufacturer to have it tested! But the medication was fine and we were left with no explanation for why my symptoms had flared so suddenly. Though all of them were common effects of MS, it was never mentioned or suspected.

Suddenly, one side of my face went numb. That got my family doctor's attention and made her think about an underlying neurological problem. She sent me to a neurologist and a subsequent MRI showed that I had several lesions on my brain. All the puzzle pieces then fell into place and nine years after the onset of symptoms I was finally diagnosed with MS.

Since then, I haven't had any more panic attacks but I've continued to struggle with my sleep and a dysfunctional bladder. I also experience crushing attacks of fatigue and my cognitive problems are worsening. My memory is poor, I can't concentrate and I don't process information as quickly as I used to. Lately I've been having episodes of vertigo that have been completely incapacitating - something I've never experienced before. (MS is an illness that keeps on giving! Just when you think you've figured it out, it presents you with something new.)

The combined effect of these impairments has been devastating - especially from a career perspective. When you're tired all the time and can't count on your sleep, it's difficult to hold down a full-time job. When you can't digest words and accurately summarize information in a timely fashion, it's impossible to work for hire as a writer.

Happily, I've found a way to remain creative and productive by sharing my own story. I wrote my book Faulty Wiring: Living with Invisible MS to draw attention to the hidden impact of MS and expand the definition of what it means to have this illness beyond mobility impairment. There are many people like me who are struggling with disabling symptoms that are imperceptible to - and misunderstood by - others and I wanted to give voice to their experience and let them know they're not alone.

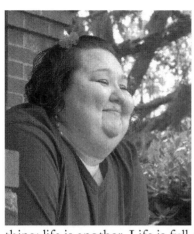

Tia Borkowski (USA)
Hit those curve balls

I had dreams when I was young. I wanted to be the next Mariah Carey or Whitney Houston or a writer or, briefly, a detective. Dreams are one thing; life is another. Life is full of curve balls. Shortly after high school my son was born.

Being the best mom to my little guy became my only dream. Through most of the following decade, I worked in customer service instead of the spotlight in smoky bars or concert venues.

The curve balls kept on coming. Just when I thought that homerun dream was in sight the umpire called another foul ball. I was finally on the path of realizing my dream as a writer when pain landed me in the emergency room. All I had to show for my dreams was myriad symptoms with no diagnosis or probable cause.

Eventually receiving the diagnosis of rheumatoid arthritis (RA) just months before my 30th birthday was the most challenging curve ball yet, or so I originally thought. Early on I was stuck in bed and in anger. I reached out on the internet for someone, anyone, who knew what I was going through and could help me make sense of it all.

One of the most helpful connections I made at that time was with a volunteer organization that provided me with friendship and resources, as well as an opportunity to work. I felt more vital and valuable, I suddenly had a purpose again! Through them, I learned what it means to be a "spoonie" (a person with chronic illness, pain or fatigue who must manage their energy consumption daily). I connected with men and women like myself, many of whom are now close friends. It didn't matter if our diseases were different we understood what it meant to have good days and bad. We could support and encourage each other!

I found my new passion, my new homerun. I may be chronically ill and in pain but I am realizing my dreams and so much more. I AM a writer, as well as a chronic illness advocate, an amateur photographer, crafter and artist. I live in the scenic Pacific Northwest where I am surrounded by beauty. I play with my Lhasa Apso, Toddy, who is both my service dog and constant companion. I support and enjoy my husband's music career, helping him chase his own dreams. I spend summers with our teenage son who makes me incredibly proud. I sell my creations on Etsy and create little packages of "happy mail" for other spoonies.

When I give back to the chronic illness community and raise awareness of our plight I am flooded with joy. I may not work a regular job but I'm far from useless. I'm a mother, a sister, a daughter, a wife. I'm a warrior, an advocate and a survivor. I still have my sense of humor. I'm at bat, hitting those curve balls right back at life!

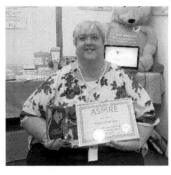

Victoria Abbott-Fleming (UK)
Life is precious

I enjoyed all that life had to offer while growing up as an only child in the North West of the United Kingdom. I loved learning, sports, music and my early school life. I was made Head Girl in primary and secondary school and later, School Prefect and Head of House. Even though I was an only child, I had many friends and was a happy youngster.

I became the first female in my family to go to university, studying for a joint honours degree of Law and Spanish. I eventually qualified as a Barrister and was called to the Bar in 2002. I loved it and knew it was a tough profession to get in but it was what I wanted to do.

I started lecturing in law. In 2003, at just 24 years old, I suffered what seemed a simple accident at work which very quickly turned complex. After seven months, I was diagnosed with a condition called complex regional pain syndrome (CRPS) in my right leg. CRPS is a rare chronic neuropathic pain condition that is thought to be the most painful chronic condition currently known.

The condition caused severe burning in my right leg, extreme sensitivity with even the most minor changes in temperature or environment and colour and temperature changes. I suffered hair loss, brittle toe nails and swelling of my leg and foot. Eventually, the skin started to breakdown from the constant swelling and ulcers developed with weeping fluid, inviting a scary experience with non-medical maggots and infection of the extremity.

I saw numerous specialists including some who told me the pain was all in my head. I tried most treatments available, including medication, regional and lumbar blocks, spinal cord stimulator, physiotherapy and more. After nearly 3 years of unsuccessful, non-stop treatments, the doctors decided that my leg needed to be amputated above the knee. I was just 27 years old with my whole future ahead of me including an excellent legal career.

It took a long time for me to accept my condition and the amputation. When I finally did, I felt that I had achieved something great and was determined that this condition was never going to beat me. Yes, I had my good days and my bad/low days but that's the way of CRPS.

Following my 1st amputation, I tried to rehabilitate onto prosthetics but it was impossible due to the CRPS (pain) remaining in my residual stump. I also experienced terrible phantom limb pain which was and still is like having the CRPS in the lower part of a leg that isn't there. I also suffered with several pneumonias and eventually contracted the complication of swine flu while on holiday in New York in January 2014.

I was given a course of ECMO and put into an induced coma for 15 days to help keep me alive. While I was in the coma, my husband was told I had less than 20% chance of survival and if I did survive, would possibly have some brain damage. I did wake up but was extremely ill. Unfortunately, after I returned to the UK new yet familiar symptoms started up.

In March 2014, I heard those fateful words, "Yes, it's definitely CRPS that's spread to your left leg." I cried. Why did it have to happen to me? What had I done to deserve this pain and suffering? A top specialist told me nothing more could be done.

After just 9 months, in late November 2014, the skin on my remaining leg started to break down and ulcerate as had the other leg. My remaining leg was amputated above the knee only 2 weeks before Christmas. The same surgeon who amputated my right leg eight years prior stood over me and told me not to worry; I was going to be okay. This second above-knee amputation left me confined to a wheelchair. I was unable to use prosthetics due to severe pain and hypersensitivity from the CRPS. I was just 35.

It was after learning about the CRPS in my left leg that my husband and I realized life was precious and short. We decided that no one should go through what we had without any form of support. I wanted to help those affected by this devastating, life-changing condition and raise awareness of it. Support and information relating to CRPS was inadequate in the UK. We had to support not only those living with

CRPS but their loved ones, families, friends and caregivers, as well. I found that most medical professionals didn't seem to be aware of this condition and they needed information. Burning Nights CRPS Support was born.

Our group provides regular blogs, an e-newsletter and a forum to help connect other sufferers along with other services including the latest research and information about all aspects of living with CRPS. You can find out more about Burning Nights CRPS Support at www.burningnightscrps.org.

I still have CRPS in both remaining stumps, as well as phantom limb pain. I do have a slightly better quality of life now, as I no longer have weeping and ulcerated legs.

Don't let anyone tell you that you can't achieve something because you can! My husband and I live by 2 quotes, "I can and I will...I can't and I won't" and "No matter how hard life is or how hard things become, don't give up. Instead, keep going because you'll get there in the end, despite the problems that life throws at you."

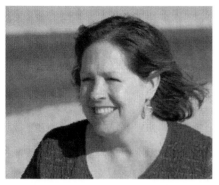

Yvonne deSousa (USA)
Defiance, with humor

I was blessed to grow up in a small town on Cape Cod, a place filled with as much beauty as its rich history, encouraging artistic vision and a vibrant tourist season. My family, friends and I found time to enjoy the beauty of our surroundings while we also worked hard. I wasn't the only local ten-year-old with my own high-end shell selling business and two part-time jobs; one as a sidewalk sweeper and the other as a mother's helper. Lucky for me, the mom I helped liked the beach. It was a great gig.

At age twelve I was the manager of my family's guesthouse and by age fourteen I had obtained a "real" job complete with paying my own small tax share to Uncle Sam. Those real jobs of my teen years consisted of candy peddling, gift shop cashiering and waitressing. The point being I knew how to work hard even before I graduated high school.

After graduating from the University of Massachusetts/Boston, I returned home for a bit to work at a local library. When volunteering at a domestic violence shelter steered me to a job working with crime victims, I went back to the city. After eight years I missed the Cape, so I returned home and took a job as an office assistant at a dental practice. That was the year I turned forty and received my diagnosis of multiple sclerosis (MS).

I was luckier than most in that I received my diagnosis in just over a month. I also had more familiarity with multiple sclerosis than the average person, as my sister had been living with it for several years. Still, the news of an incurable, debilitating, chronic illness was quite the blow and as I had been battling extreme fatigue for so long I just didn't know how I could handle the MS beast. I was easily frustrated with the craziness that life with MS was throwing at me and needed a means to manage that craziness. It was then that I started using my sense of humor to write about the "crazy" in a sense, beating on the MS bully.

Several months later, cognitive difficulties forced me to quit my job. Vocational counseling and research in the want ads did little to help me figure out how I would support myself. Not working was not something I could foresee in my life; I had been working since I was ten! My neurologist thought it best if I only worked part-time, yet a part-time job wouldn't provide affordable insurance. More frustration, more MS crazy. The more frustrations took hold, the more I had to write about them to feel like I was fighting back and at least doing something.

Before I knew it, I had the start of a book, a memoir designed to make people laugh at my expense. Would this work? Could I become a writer? Would people care what I had to say? Could I support myself that way?

I joined a writing group and realized the joy that comes from laughter. Whenever members of my group, my friends or fellow writers at open mic nights laughed at my work, it made them happy and it inspired me. Before long, I had a successful blog and just over two years later, MS Madness! A "Giggle More, Cry Less" Story of Multiple Sclerosis was published. Immediately MS Madness! began receiving rave reviews and endorsements, including this one from Richard M. Cohen, NY Times best-selling author of Blindsided and Strong at the Broken Places: "MS Madness! A 'Giggle More, Cry Less' Story of Multiple Sclerosis combines defiance with humor, the secret weapon of the sick."

In those years before the release of MS Madness!, as I was pursuing a career in writing, I had my essays published in several places, including Chicken Soup for the Soul: Finding My Faith, Something on Our Minds Volumes 1-3, CapeWomenOnline, the Cape Cod Times and the Provincetown Banner. Additionally, a Christian play I wrote titled The Best Birthday Ever has been performed in over six countries and translated into Spanish.

While I don't know if I can call my published works a career, they are an excellent incentive for me to keep writing, moving forward and to keep smiling. More importantly, my writing is making others smile, too. That is my deepest joy.

If you need a giggle today, check out my website, yvonnedesousa.com, where you will find my blog, my book and "Laugh Lines" -one-liners from people, famous and not-so-famous, designed to provide an instant smile.

PART 2 - How We Learned to Live Well with Chronic Illness and Disability

Chapter 1
The Devastation and Delight of Diagnosis

My Advice For The Newly-Diagnosed With ME/CFS
By Miranda Brewster

(Editor's note: Much of Miranda's advice will help anyone with any chronic illness.)

I've had ME (myalgic encephalomyelitis, also known as chronic fatigue syndrome) since 2001 and over the years I've learned what to do and what not to do with this illness. I'd like to share some of my experience with you:

1. When you receive your diagnosis, don't panic! It's a horrible illness but it can be managed.
2. Always get new symptoms checked out by a doctor to eliminate other conditions.
3. If your GP isn't particularly supportive, you can change GP's. You may be referred to an ME/CFS clinic, which may or may not give you good advice. You need to do what you feel will be helpful and don't be pushed or bullied; it's your body!
4. Social services may be able to help you with your needs.
5. Educate yourself about the illness as much as possible.
   a. Here are some books written by ME/CFS sufferers that I recommend. Sufferers tend to know more about the experience of this illness than the medical profession, so it's helpful to seek their advice
      i. Severe ME/CFS: A Guide to Living by Emily Collingridge
      ii. Fighting Fatigue: A practical guide to managing the symptoms of CFS/ME edited by Sue Pemberton and Catherine Berry
      iii. 101 Tips for Coping with ME by Hayley Green (good for the newly diagnosed)
      iv. My A-Z of M.E. by Ros Lemarchand (poetry about living with ME)
   b. Seek out ME/CFS support groups; there are loads of them, including a few groups on Facebook. In the UK, the ME Association is

helpful in finding a local support group for you and offers other valuable information.

c. Search for blogs and vlogs on the internet about ME/CFS. I find Barry's M.E. Blog and his YouTube channel to be informative. YouTube is full of videos with useful information about ME and you can feel free to contact these people. I've found them more than willing to help. Two other blogs I like are Pajama Daze, and M.E. myself and I. My husband has ME, too, so he and I created our own website called Dozy Dayz, offering advice, links and videos about ME.

d. Another useful educational tool is the dvd, Voices from the Shadows, which is available to view for free on Vimeo. It highlights severe ME. Don't let the severity of this illness as it is portrayed in this video frighten you. Not everyone with ME gets this ill but it's a good tool to handout to GP's, family and friends to educate and help them support you.

6. You may hear negative comments about your condition. It's good to have a prepared response so you feel more in control and able to educate those who are ill-informed.

7. Be wary of those who profess to have instant cures, particularly those that cost a fortune, because there are no cures. Instead, look for recovery stories, like <u>Why ME? My Journey from M.E. to Health and Happiness</u> by Alex Howard. Be open-minded, as everybody's ME/CFS is different. What works for one may not work for another. Don't dismiss someone's recovery story. Look outside the box; their methods may be worth a try. This disease needs to be dealt with from many different angles.

8. Prepare for bad days. Stock up on easy meals that require little preparation. Put together a "First Aid Kit" by filling a box with things like cheery dvds, a list of

people for support, little journals, coloring books, music, etc.

9. We need to do more of what is helpful and less of what is unhelpful; this includes being around positive, helpful people and avoiding those who are negative or unhelpful.

10. Learn to relax. That's difficult to do when we feel dreadful and life is uncertain. Relaxation improves digestion and it helps to stabilize our symptoms. We can learn to relax with books like <u>Relaxation for Dummies</u> by Shamash Alidina and other relaxation cds, dvds and videos on YouTube and those available to purchase online or on demand.

11. Nurture yourself with a regular schedule of rest, good nutrition, and a calm environment. ME/CFS responds well to routine, so create a schedule with light activity and relaxation. Pace yourself and show yourself compassion. It's time to put yourself first!

Diagnosis: MS! My Initial Reaction
By Yvonne Desousa

My initial reactions to my relapsing-remitting multiple sclerosis diagnosis were about as varied as the initial symptoms themselves. But they primarily came down to five-

1. I can't stay in the hospital; Christmas is next week!
2. Are you sure that big blob on my brain scan is not a tumor? 'Cause it really, really looks like a tumor.' (And, of course, I would know because I have zero medical experience and barely passed biology in high school.)
3. So...I'm not a hypochondriac, insane, or suffering from early onset Alzheimer's disease? Then I guess MS is okay.
4. Can I use this diagnosis to get out of work tomorrow?
5. And finally, (and I guess this was my overall reaction that I was desperately trying to push to the back of my lesion-filled brain): Holy ****! I have MS!

Reaction #1 was born of the unusual set of circumstances that lead to my diagnosis in the first place. That morning I stumbled into work on my numb and tingling legs. (Here is part of the chronic illness crazy: how could my legs be numb AND tingly? If they were numb, I couldn't feel them. How did I know they were tingly? But they were and I did.) I knew it was going to be busy at the dentist office where I worked; clean teeth for mistletoe kisses are very important. I didn't expect much else to take place. True, I had just undergone a series of MRI's to determine what was going on with my legs, but the technologists were vague about when I would get the results. Yet only a few hours into the day my primary care doctor called and told me I had MS. I needed to immediately get to a hospital (over 90 miles away) where the head of neurology would squeeze me in for an evaluation, if I could get there in the next few hours.

"And be prepared to stay," she added to this already overwhelming information.

Be prepared to stay at a hospital? How does one prepare for that? Should I go home (30 miles in the opposite direction) and pack a bag? What does one pack? A toothbrush, I guess. I worked for a dentist; I could grab a toothbrush here. Socks? Yes, definitely socks. Cold feet drive me crazy. A book? Yes, a book would be good. But I wouldn't have time to read; Christmas was next week! Should I pack all the Christmas cards I still had to write? How about all the Christmas presents I still had to wrap? Should I bring presents, bows, tape and paper with me?

In the end, I skipped the "prepare to stay" part and just got on the highway. As it turned out, I didn't need to stay, which freed my mind to focus on other things. Like the scan this neurologist I had never met showed me. Apparently, MS is hard to diagnosis in many people. In my case, to the trained eye, MULTIPLE SCLEROSIS was practically written across my skull in the gadolinium used to highlight the lesions. All I saw was a scary looking blob. "Are you sure that's not a brain tumor? Cause it really, really looks like a brain tumor!" Once the doctor explained the difference between MS lesions and brain tumors, I felt a little better.

Then I began to realize that I hadn't been crazy when I described to my friends the weird things going on in my body. We had decided that these things - having to pee constantly, the fatigue, weird sudden sharp pains, the crankiness, the fatigue, the temperature sensitivity, the abdominal pain and did I mention the fatigue - were the result of aging. We also decided that because they bothered me so much, I must be a whiner. The early symptoms that concerned me the most were the extreme spacey brain and memory difficulties I was experiencing. My grandmother had Alzheimer's but she was in her seventies. I was only forty. What would my life be like if I was getting Alzheimer's now? Being told that these issues were due to MS was a relief! I understood that MS wouldn't be a picnic but it seemed less threatening than Alzheimer's.

As the appreciation of one serious illness over another took effect, my mind drifted to ways to use this news to my advantage. I now knew I didn't have to stay in the hospital but I really did still have a lot to do in the next few days and I was so very tired. (Have I mentioned the horrible fatigue?) Could I use my diagnosis as an excuse to call in sick at work the next morning?

As it turns out, I could. The neurologist scheduled steroid infusions for the next several days to start treatment. Luckily, I could do them at a hospital closer to me and yes, I would need to miss work for the very first one.

Though some of this news was good (I didn't have Alzheimer's and I got to miss work the next day), it was still a lot to take in. I was only just starting to process the diagnosis and scary emotions (panic, dread, sorrow) careened in my blob-filled brain. As the information began to settle there was one reaction left; the most obvious reaction of all. I was stumbling out of the hospital when it hit.

HOLY ****! I HAVE MS!

Diagnosis And Divorce
By Mary Pettigrew

I was diagnosed with multiple sclerosis (MS) in July of 2001. At first, the opinion was "maybe" I had multiple sclerosis or transverse myelitis. After a rough recuperation from a bad reaction to the lumbar puncture a third neurologist/neuro surgeon confirmed it as definitely MS. In all honesty, I was calm and relieved when the doctor told me. Or maybe it was shock or denial. I'm not sure. I certainly had no idea as to what was in store for me in the coming years.

My family and friends were very sad, yet supportive. My father flew in from California to "hold my paw" as he lovingly says. My brother cried as I told him over the phone; he now tells me it's because he knew someone who had a friend who died from MS. We know that MS itself isn't a death sentence but death can occur from complications from the disease, or from the additional autoimmune diseases and syndromes people sometimes acquire. I do have a handful of additional autoimmune issues but do my best to carry on.

After receiving my diagnosis and weaning off heavy steroids, I took several weeks off from my job as catering director for a high end (and VERY busy) private dining club in Fort Worth. Once I returned to work, things seemed "business as usual" for a while and I maintained my reputation as reliable and competent. After the 9/11 attacks, I began to tire much faster and I started making mistakes, forgetting details for various events. I became moody and more sensitive to stress, which led to more time off and debilitating fatigue.

My managers and co-workers had no idea how to handle me and they feared I was now a detriment to the establishment. I assume they had studied up on the ADA rules and to avoid violation of those rules, they "kindly" found ways to make me so miserable that I'd quit. In 2002, I did. I continued to bounce back and forth between taking time off and attempting jobs with less responsibility, yet I couldn't handle them and took many sick days. I would always quit each job before facing the risk of getting fired.

A couple of exacerbations popped up between my original diagnosis and quitting work for good. In 2005, it was time to file for SSDI. After denials and appeals and a lawyer, I was approved. The judge deemed me to be disabled as of December 2002. That was great news! The back pay I received was a much-needed boost, yet my husband (now ex-husband) took quite a bit of it for his own purposes without telling me. That was a tell-tale sign of things yet to come in our marriage. Our relationship grew more and more distant, almost as if we were living as roommates instead of husband and wife. He became increasingly embarrassed by my illness and how it affected HIS lifestyle.

Long story short, for several years I wanted out but I feared how I would survive financially. One day I woke up and decided enough was enough. The life I was living was a farce and to be alone and struggling financially was a better option than where I was at that time. I was merely existing day to day and I knew it was time to file for divorce in 2009. The next 6 years were a battle - the stories deserve a book of their own- but I survived. I'm still here and I'm living my life.

Digesting My Diagnosis
By Melanie Styles

I sat in my nurse practitioner's office anxiously awaiting her arrival. Here I am, her Problem Patient; the one who always has something wrong, the fibromyalgia patient, the depressed hypochondriac. I have never been diagnosed by a psychiatric professional as clinically depressed. It's just a term that medical doctors used whenever I cried from frustration, because they weren't helping me. I wasn't a hypochondriac. Eventually my complaints proved to be medically sound, once the doctors admitted that they had no idea what was going on with my body and dug a little deeper.

She walked in. Here we go again.

"Do you hear that?" I asked.

"Yes," she said. "What is that?"

"It's the roof of my mouth. You know, between my nose and my mouth. It keeps going up and down and it makes that noise."

"You're not doing that on purpose?"

I shook my head. She walked closer and noticed that my throat was moving, then had me open my mouth. When I did, the noise stopped but my soft palate was still moving rhythmically. She went to get a couple more nurses and another doctor to observe it. She thought maybe I had a sinus infection because she had just treated two of my children for infections the week before. She innocently threw antibiotics at me thinking mucus was moving around in my sinus cavity.

After two weeks, the rhythmic clicking did not stop. As you can imagine, any noise that you hear 24/7can drive you a crazy. This is somewhat like tinnitus in that respect but others hear it, too! I got tired of answering questions such as, "Are you doing that on purpose?" and "Does it hurt?" I was keeping myself awake at night. If it were my husband having this problem, I would've smothered him in his sleep. (I'm sure he'd have wanted it that way.)

I made an appointment with an ear, nose and throat doctor (ENT). In the meantime, I searched online to see what could possibly be causing the clicking and what solutions could be found. I went through a very similar conversation with the ENT to the one I had with my general practitioner. He looked in my mouth, left the room and came back with another doctor. He had a look on his face as if he had seen a ghost.

He said, "You have palatal myoclonus (PM). It is a very rare seizure disorder; hard to treat. It is usually treated with anti-seizure medications but I don't feel comfortable treating it. You should see a neurologist."

This was the first time I ever had a doctor state that he was not knowledgeable enough to treat my condition.

It is worth noting that I did have a neurologist who felt he was capable of treating both my fibromyalgia and my palatal myoclonus but I disagreed with his methodology. Instead of listening to my symptoms and my issues, he heard "fibromyalgia patient" and "palatal myoclonus patient" and treated me based on research. When I read my patient notes, he had not been recording my weekly symptoms as I reported them and had been misreporting my progress making it appear that I was responding to the medications better than I was.

I told a couple close friends and family members I had this rare condition called PM and described it to them. In each case they said, "I know someone who has that in their jaw." I had to explain it is not TMJ. It is not my jaw. It is my soft palate. I'm starting to believe that people do not understand the word "rare." If everyone knows someone who has a disease, then by definition, it is not rare. I explain to people that not all seizures are epileptic or grand mal. As a teacher, I feel we've failed society.

While I was digesting it all, I remember feeling weird. I knew I should have felt horrible about my diagnosis because of my doctor's shocked reaction but I didn't. When talking to people about it, they kept apologizing and that didn't bother me. Maybe I was numb; by this point I had already been through so much, health-wise. I knew that there was something seriously wrong with me neurologically for quite some time but doctors were dismissive about it. Now that I had a diagnosis for this seizure disorder, the doctors could no longer ignore it.

I have settled into my PM. While I'm still searching for a neurologist who will listen and care enough to find the cause of the illness and cure me, I am not scrambling for a cure. I am quietly frustrated because I believe with all my strength that the secret to all my illness lies in my brain. I believe my PM is my brain crying out, "Listen to me, please!"

Chapter 2
Emotions, Changes and Suffering

Learning To Laugh At The MS Bully
By Yvonne Desousa

The one part of my body that refuses to be attacked by multiple sclerosis is my funny bone. Because of that fact, I'm still sane.

Sure, you're probably thinking this doesn't make sense since our bodies don't really contain a "funny bone." As little about chronic illness makes sense, I'm depending on the strength and fierceness of my own personal funny bone and using it to beat the crap out of multiple sclerosis (MS)!

Who could have possibly thought that an inappropriate comment after my MS diagnosis would lead to a new sense of humor? The speaker of the comment was my little brother, Chris, who had driven me to the hospital. Hours later when we were walking out of the building he said, "You know, you can totally get one of those handicapped parking plates now."

I thought his comment was a sincere attempt at finding the good in the bad in a "this really sucks but at least there's this" kind of way. Parking was the last thing on my mind and I told him so. He responded, "Even if you don't want to use it right away you could let me borrow it."

The kid was a twenty-one-year-old semi-pro dirt bike rider who drove a huge Ford F150 pickup truck with two dirt bikes in the bed. I pictured him behind the wheel of his gargantuan vehicle backing into a handicapped spot and I was laughing hysterically. It helped.

People told me it was okay to be angry about my diagnosis. They insisted that I should be angry. They questioned why I wasn't angry. "Are you sure you have MS? You don't seem very angry." I think I was too tired to be angry. What I was, was frustrated. How could I not be angry as I learned more about this illness that had already caused me so much grief? The horrific "my-entire-insides-twisting-as-if-in-a-vise" stomach ache that I used as an excuse to not eat my vegetables; that nightmare was called a hug. An MS hug. Who came up with that??

My new interferon injections were made from Chinese hamster ovary cells. I now had to inject myself with this medication that cost ten times as much as my paycheck and it was made from hamsters? Why hamsters? Why not goldfish? Or guinea pigs? Why not parakeets? And why was it so damn expensive? Last I knew hamsters were pretty cheap. Perhaps if I went to China, brought back a few and started breeding them, I could get a discount?

Speaking of prescription costs, what could I do but laugh manically at the case worker from my insurance company who called to say she was assigned to help me with the stress of living with a chronic illness but who refused to discuss why my co-pays went from $3.65 to $2200 in one month?

"I can't help you with financial matters," she told me. "I'm here to help you cope with the stress of living with MS. Do you have any stress from living with MS?"

"I'm completely stressed about how I'm going to pay these ridiculous co-pays for my MS medication."

"But that's not what I'm here for. Let me send you some pamphlets on coping with stress. I'm sure those will help."

Then there was the pharmacist who filled my entire stimulant prescription (legal speed) with no problem but would only dispense two prescription vitamin D pills at a time because he was afraid I might abuse them.

It became clear that life with a chronic illness was going to be insane. I was already having cognitive problems and didn't need to add insanity to the mix. I thought back to how laughing at Chris' comment on the day of my diagnosis was such a great stress reliever; way better than any pamphlet the insurance people sent me. To make me laugh more, I started making fun of the crazy and it helped me feel better. For example:

> MS comes with fatigue. Fatigue causes increased loss of dexterity. Eating healthy may help combat the fatigue. Eating healthy involves vegetables which involve chopping and dicing. So, let's give a tired, clumsy girl an onion and a sharp knife and tell her it's good for her.

> Water is good for you; you need to drink lots of water. An overactive bladder is a huge problem for some people with MS (like me). You can take medication to help with your bladder but that medication causes wicked dry mouth. The cure for dry

mouth is drinking more water. My choice seemed to be to expound on this phenomenon in a humorous way or permanently move into my bathroom.

Exercise is also good for you; it will help give you energy. But you need energy to exercise! What comes first? Energy or exercise? Trying to understand this chronic illness dilemma kept me on my sofa for hours thinking about it.

There are plenty of statistics that say a positive attitude is good for well-being. What can be more positive than a smile, a giggle or an all-out hysterical belly laugh born out of a vicious attempt at making fun of the MS bully? No, MS isn't funny. With the right perspective and a strong funny bone, I argue that life with MS can be a freaking riot!

Survivor Seeking Serenity: A 12-Year Journey
By Katherine Dunn

June 21st, 2017 marked the 12-year anniversary of the day I injured my back. I live in constant pain, somehow manage to keep my head above water and usually have a smile on my face.

The best gift chronic pain gave me was my jewelry; making this helps me survive the pain. Just designing pieces in my head makes me happy and surprisingly proud. I am thrilled to have gained the expertise to develop my own unique style and a creative outlet that distracts me effectively from the pain.

I thought I had it all figured out. Then our son moved back home in Fall 2016.

For some reason his return triggered panic attacks - perplexing, as he was so helpful. He remembered to ask if I needed anything, opened my blinds when I woke and picked up items I dropped. He seems to understand my pain in a very real sense. What was wrong? My anxiety grew.

Come January, I was exhausted. Finding the energy to move felt impossible. By February, life was a constant panic attack. It took all my coping techniques to survive. I have never felt the need to watch so much comedy! The anxiety was subsiding but the depression was not.

I decided to make my husband's birthday in April a special day. It quickly became a comedy of errors. I had to climb our stairs three times in one day - stairs I normally climbed twice a WEEK!

I took a bath and ordered takeout.

The next day I tried to get up and fell back on the bed. When I stood the pain was unbearable. An hour later, I took pain meds and tried again with my cane. I managed to get to my walker by leaning on my cane and furniture.

The struggle continued. All my energy went into trying to walk, putting most of my weight on my hands. It was three weeks before I could take more than two steps unaided. The feeling of desperation was growing. I was only going upstairs for a bath every five days. It took every ounce of my strength to convince myself to climb those stairs.

Eventually all the rest, stretches, restorative yoga and massage led to progress. Five weeks later, I was able to walk mostly unaided inside the house but still had not recovered completely.

Those five weeks dragged at my soul. I had spent the past four years avoiding thoughts of the future. I couldn't hide from it any longer. It was glaringly obvious that I couldn't depend on my ability to walk.

Luckily, my home was small and I had chairs or stools in every single room. I stopped and rested often. Unfortunately, all my efforts, tricks and assistive devices simply weren't enough. As long as we had stairs, I risked a flare that could ruin my life for weeks. What if I didn't recover from the next one? It seemed that I would never be able to breathe easy again. The anxiety was overwhelming.

Early in June, it hit me. The reason for my desperation, the root of my depression and anxiety was this: I needed hope for the future!

I had been living in a studio flat in the basement to make things easier for me. It was large and everything I needed was there. Before Simon moved back in, I had intended to move upstairs. We had planned to relocate the living room to our bedroom and the office to Simon's old room. It wasn't a clear plan but it was a plan. With Simon in the house that plan couldn't work. I had lost my hope.

I realized what I needed was assurance that I could move upstairs permanently if I could no longer climb the stairs. I had to figure out the minimum space needed, not only to survive but to keep me moderately happy. I could finally fall asleep when I created a plan for an 8x9 foot room off the kitchen.

I woke with a renewed sense of purpose and without the cloud of desperation! I had a plan! Not the best one but one I knew we could manage. Bathing when I wanted, going out on the balcony to sit in the sun, boiling water and making toast at the same time and eating with my family.

Yet as tempting as it sounded, I realized I liked my life as it was.

I love my big room downstairs where I have space for my jewelry supplies. I enjoy my sit-in kitchenette, my bedroom with everything I need in one place and my tiny bathroom that I didn't have to share.

I choose to live downstairs but now I have a plan that can work! I realized that just like a doomsday bunker the new room wouldn't be a place to live full-time until absolutely necessary; it is an escape plan, reassuring me that my future is secure. With this new perspective I feel content and have a new appreciation for my reality!

It's incredible how hope and freedom of choice are so important to our survival. I choose to move forward and NOT focus on all I have lost, on the daily struggles, nor on the fact that my life feels like training for a marathon, while it looks like I do nothing.

I miss a great deal living with chronic pain but most days my life feels full and rewarding. And the other days? They don't last forever. After 12 years, that's the best lesson I have learned. Life is a rollercoaster. There are many ups and downs, and surprise twists and turns. Nothing ever stays the same. Intense pain dulls, muscle spasms calm, sadness turns to smiles and you can always choose to make the best of it. Just throw your hands up and let out a cry of joy when you're on top. Enjoy every single second.

My Treatise On Fear (Or Is This My Treaty With Fear?)
By Cameron Auxer

(first published in My Journal on Inspire.com under 2young4this)

One night I broke down. Nights can be the darkest time for me; it is quiet and I hear my thoughts, loud and clear. I cried hard and long that dark night without a sound, so as not to disturb the other tenants. What I thought was grief emerged from the marrow of my bones and came out as a silent scream. As my tears subsided, I suddenly realized that it wasn't as much grief, or anger, or sadness that I was experiencing. It was fear.

All negative emotions stem from fear. What was I afraid of?

I thought back to when I had been diagnosed with cancer requiring surgery in 2002, living in a foreign land with no family or friends nearby. People said I was brave. But I was frightened; courage had nothing to do with it. I faced a situation where I had little choice.

I remembered that the prospect of death was not what frightened me at the time. Maybe I was afraid of suffering, yes. What scared me the most was LIFE! I was alone and all the possibilities of life were daunting. I had no companion. My friends lived hours or days away. Though my parents sent inspiring emails from afar, other family members never called, emailed or asked how I was doing. I was scared that I was unlovable.

I lived through years of heart attacks, migraines and dizziness, fatigue and the threat of stroke and arterial dissection. My arthritis continued to spread painfully. My short-term memory became a patchwork quilt with many frayed pieces. The fear continued to rear its ugly head.

Scared of becoming a lonely, feeble old woman. Scared of being in pain, having a stroke, suffering more heart attacks, getting slammed again by fatigue and being unable to care for myself, with no one to help me. Scared of people thinking I'm a fraud. Scared of being abandoned by those who say they love me. Scared of losing good medical care. Scared that I'd never be the dynamic, energetic person I once was. Scared that I'd forget how to laugh and love.

None of us wants to suffer. However, the fear of pain can be even worse than the pain itself. The fear of pain is the fertile ground where suffering arises. If pain does happen, the suffering grows because we don't believe the pain will ever end. My fear of LIFE would certainly keep me in pain - emotional pain.

Remembering the quote by Franklin D. Roosevelt, "Only thing we have to fear is fear itself," I started to ponder what fear really was. I realized it was nothing. Absolutely nothing. It was a self-manufactured non-entity that kept me from living life fully and somehow I needed to find a way to embrace the unknown without it.

My lovely book of Prayers for Healing (Conari Press, 1997, M. Oman, ed., p. 114) offered a bit of wisdom, excerpted from A Course in Miracles. It talked about how the only way we can face reality is to stare our illusions right in the face. We should not be afraid, for when we face our illusions we are looking at our "source of fear" and it is then that we gain the knowledge that "fear is not real."

Ah ha.

Yep, I still have fears. There are all sorts of creepy crawlies inside my head that I've clung to ever since "something happened," I decided "it was bad" and "I don't want it to happen again." I'm working on it. I realize that all that stuff is just a bunch of "What ifs?". The bad stuff may happen. Then again, maybe it won't.

LIFE happens every second of every day for as long as we take a breath. There is no way for us to know what each moment will bring. To live in fear of the future based on our experience of the past, eliminates the possibility of experiencing joy in the present. Oh, how I want to choose joy. I may have to continually remind myself to make that choice. But I do want it. I want it bad.

Chapter 3
Self-Care and Creating Balance

Creating Balance: Making Room For Joy In Your Life
By Cameron Auxer

(first published in My Journal on Inspire.com under 2young4this)

Perhaps you work, have a family, belong to a church or group...and you have chronic illness. Illness comes with its own set of requirements: doctor appointments, taking medications, surgeries, special diets. Illness is work. We work twice as hard as anyone just to get out of bed. We may juggle a full life but with illness and fatigue the balls eventually start to drop. The house is in chaos. The boss threatens to fire you for being late. The kids whine for attention. Your spouse can't understand why you aren't "in the mood."

There's a saying that goes like this: "Tend to the well. If it runs dry, no one gets a drink." This applies to you, your body, your life. Tend to it. This may go against your grain as you may feel it's your duty to put others' needs first. But if your well runs dry, if you become bedridden with exhaustion, how can you care for anyone else?

"BUT," you say, "They need me!"

Examine your feeling of guilt. Self-care is not selfish. When life is balanced you can better control your environment and create a space that is nurturing and stable. Happy, secure people face crises with more strength than those who sabotage their health and live on the edge. Why feel guilty about making life better for yourself and everyone you love?

If there is imbalance in your life, if demands outweigh your self-care, then something's gotta give! You must accept that you cannot and do not have to do it all yourself! Small children can put away toys. Children over the age of four can make beds and tidy their rooms. School age children can put away laundry and help with dishes, house cleaning and yard work. Teens can also plan meals, do laundry, mow the lawn and babysit. Older teens can chauffeur, as well. Spouses can certainly help with cooking, cleanup and other duties, too.

You are NOT taking away your children's childhood. You are teaching them responsibility along with respect for your situation. Hold a family meeting and negotiate as to who will do what. A chore chart can be posted as a reminder. Delegate with a smile, provide reward, make it fun and enjoy raising a responsible, self-efficient family. (Your children's future spouses will love you for it!) Create balance by allowing ample time for everyone to play and relax together, alone or with friends. This is where the joy comes in!

If you live alone, friends can be marvelous help. Discuss your limitations so they understand your needs. Ask if they can run an errand for you or assist you one day per week. Barter in exchange for help. My friend assists me with gardening, repairs and shopping. I share meals with him.

Simplify your life. Get rid of clutter. Clean out book shelves and buy e-readers. Give away items that aren't used and clothes that aren't worn. With less mess your family can streamline their cleaning routine.

If you must work or if you choose to keep working, then scrutinize whether your current job is the best fit for you. Consider a less-demanding job, one that can be job-shared or that lets you work at home or part-time. Or explore adjusting your job to better suit your energy. If you choose to cut your hours, look at your finances to consider where you can cut expenses and create a budget that allows you to live well with less money.

Above all, get good at saying "No." Once you educate people on your limitations you'll find that gently and firmly declining a request or invitation is usually received with grace. Boundaries are essential.

Change doesn't happen overnight. It takes time to scale down your responsibilities and demands. Kids may rebel. So may your spouse. Be clear about your needs, kindly request cooperation and negotiate until there is agreement. Then shower them with gratitude!

Some things in life cannot be changed. You may be a caregiver. Perhaps you're a single parent. It comes down to the Serenity Prayer: Change the things you can change, accept the things you can't and have the wisdom to know the difference. Perhaps you can't change your job but you can eat healthier food, rest while the kids do chores and ask a friend to water your garden. Make changes that nurture you.

Allow the Lessons of the Well to become ingrained in your thinking and soon Balance will nourish the Joy in your life!

Creating A Healing Space
By Abbie Levy

As someone with chronic illness, I know what it's like to be stuck in pajamas, in bed or on a couch. As an Interior Designer, I am very aware of how our environment impacts how we feel. Allow me to let you in on some sound advice so you can create a healing space in your home – a place just for you to feel comforted, nurtured and even entertained during your extended down time. A place that reflects who you are and what makes you happy. A special, comfortable place for you that does not cost a lot to create!

Colors can impact your mood and feelings. To what colors are you drawn? Are there particular colors in nature that attract you? Notice the colors currently in your home and your closet. Which colors make you the happiest? Which colors calm you? If there are colors that you really love but they don't look good <u>on</u> you then enjoy having them <u>around</u> you in your new space!

Every color has properties that can support your well-being. Green can calm you. Blue is serene and aids in tranquility. Purple can put you in a romantic mood. Bright yellow can cheer you up and orange is powerful for lifting you out of despair. The most intense color is red which can stimulate your appetite and your heart rate. You may respond differently to a color than someone else would so sample the rainbow for what makes you feel best.

It's great if you can get someone to paint your room with a new color but that isn't necessary. You can add color to your space with garden flowers or artwork. If you find it difficult to cut flowers or care for plants, don't overlook the many life-like, care-free artificial plants and flowers now available. Sometimes a colorful vase of flowers is all you need to add cheer to a room!

Artwork doesn't have to be expensive. Use an inexpensive frame to feature children's art, posters or greeting cards. In a frame they will look like a masterpiece!

Pillows are a multi-functional accessory; they add splashes of color to your space, as well as provide comfort and support. Pillows are easy to make; if you are handy with a sewing machine, make your own from scarves, linens or fabric scraps!

Do you collect books by a favorite author or beautiful coffee table books full of photos of a favorite hobby or subject? Give them a special spot in your healing space. Photo albums make a great addition, as well, so you can revisit fond memories. Include whatever makes you smile; it's YOUR space!

Instead of going out to buy furniture for your space, see if there is something old in storage that can be made new again! Or check out a used furniture store. Ask a friend to help refinish an old cupboard. Use throw covers or re-cover seat cushions with fabric remnants. If your budget can handle some new furniture, buy pieces that are multipurpose, such as a day bed or storage ottoman. Or rearrange your current furniture for a new look and more functional setting.

Your healing space can be set up in your bedroom, a spare room or that little nook in your family room. Wherever you choose, be sure the location is practical. If your mobility is limited or if you will spend most of your day there, make sure the necessary facilities and much-used items are easily accessible. Organization and planning are key here. Use shoe boxes, plastic bins, laundry baskets, totes, baskets and buckets to help you keep things handy and organized. Be sure to utilize those wonderful walls around you, too! A few easy-to-reach shelves give you lots of extra storage space.

A little planning and a touch of imagination will magically create a cozy space that is uniquely you…a special place where function, accessibility and comfort come together in an oh-so-lovely and healing way!

Wrangling Medications
By Lene Andersen

Medications are your friend.

Does that sound wrong? It's a natural impulse to try to become as healthy as possible when you've been diagnosed with a chronic illness. For many this means an instinctive rejection of medication — all those chemicals can't possibly be good for you, right? We come by this opinion honestly. Despite the pervasive presence of medication in drugstores and commercials, we are taught to resist taking meds unless absolutely necessary.

These beliefs can really bite you in the butt.

Having a chronic illness means that something has gone wonky in your body. Regardless of the cause — and we don't know the cause of many chronic illnesses — the "chronic" implies that it can't be cured. Although making lifestyle changes may improve your general health and bring relief to some, for many of us it doesn't work.

Enter medications.

Taking care of yourself

When you live with chronic illness, it's extra important to take care of yourself. Self-care can take many forms including getting the rest you need, eating a healthy balanced diet, meditating, physical therapy, using hot and cold packs and taking medication.

Medications can prevent the disease from wreaking havoc on your body and they can help you feel better. They can make the difference between being stuck in bed or being able to live your life. Medications can enable you to be an active part of your family, your work, your community.

Some medications can be viewed with a stigma. Opioid painkillers have been the target of restrictive legislation and the people who need them to function are increasingly viewed with suspicion. For people who have high levels of chronic pain, opioids are simply a tool that enables them to live their lives most often without addiction. A meta-study showed that when these drugs are prescribed and taken correctly, opioid addiction rates are a quarter of one percent.[1] That means over ninety-nine percent of people who take opioid painkillers will not get addicted. This is a handy statistic to share with people who express concern that you're taking these "terrible" drugs.

Finding the right medication for you

No medication is an automatic fit for everyone and finding the one that works for you can involve trial and error. When you find the right medication it can seem like a miracle. Getting there can be a frustrating journey: waiting to see if a particular drug works, trying drugs that don't work and enduring drugs with side effects that make you feel like crap.

Most medications have a recommended dose and most doctors will prescribe that dose. This may not be right for you. Some people are sensitive to medication and need to start with less, slowly building up to a dose that works. Others need more than what is recommended. As you talk about medication options with your doctor, it's a good idea to also discuss whether you can build some flexibility into taking the medication. Most doctors will work with you if it can be done safely.

What to do about side effects

One of the common fears when taking a new medication is the potential for side effects. If you Google the drug, chances are you'll find yourself hyperventilating into a paper bag. Anytime you look up a medication you will find a list of side effects. That list includes all the possible side effects that were found in testing the drug and it can make for anxious reading. Keep in mind that just because the side effects have happened to some people in the past, doesn't mean they will happen to you. It's also important to remember that the really scary list you find under the heading of Rare Side Effects are truly rare. For most, side effects tend to be manageable.

How you deal with side effects depends on what they are and what kind of chronic illness you have. Some ways to deal with side effects include: adjusting your medication schedule, adapting what you eat and adding over-the-counter meds.

---

[1] M. Noble, et al., "Long-term opioid management for chronic noncancer pain," Cochrane Database of Systematic Reviews 1. January 20, 2010): CD006605

Sometimes it's about learning to live with a side effect because the beneficial effects of the drugs outweigh the annoyance. For instance, the medication I take for my rheumatoid arthritis gives me a lot of gas. It also controls my disease. I have learned to be a lot more relaxed about being windy. After all, the average person farts 14 times a day – who cares if I double that?

Unfortunately, there are times when the side effects may take over. If they sneak up on you, slowly building to a nasty crescendo, you may not notice at first how much they are affecting your quality of life. Then it hits you one day and that means it's time to reconsider. Medication is supposed to help you not impact your life as much — or more — as untreated illness. We all have a different line in the sand for what's a tolerable side effect and what isn't. Careful reflection will show you where your line is. If the negative effects of your medication have moved past that line, it's time to talk to your doctor about options.

At the end of the day, you must approach the treatment of your disease in a way that makes sense to you. For some that means not taking medications. For others, medications are very much part of their treatment regimen. Arriving at a decision that works for you and your disease can take a lot of thinking and discussion with your doctors. Taking the lead in managing your disease and your medications is an empowering experience, one that will help you to live better with your chronic illness.

Spending Quality Time With Kids
By Louise Bibby

Being a mother with chronic illness and pain means juggling the management of my health with being the best Mum I can. I wrote my eBook 15 Minute Power Plays with Your Kids: How to Be a Better Parent in 15 Minutes a Day because: (1) as parents we feel a lot of guilt that is often unwarranted (especially when chronically ill) and (2) often I overestimated the quality time my daughter wanted or needed with me to feel satisfied. The eBook was written for a wider audience, but as a person who has been a parent with chronic illness, most of my ideas in the book are helpful for us.

The book was written as a jog-your-memory book, like a recipe book. It's not that you don't know how to do these things, it's just that the ideas sometimes don't come to mind. The following are edited excerpts.

5 Easy 15 Minute Power Plays for Chronically Ill Parents

1. Play make-believe (Age 1 – 9) I'm amazed at how much joy it gives my daughter when I join in one of her games. I remember in the early years playing in her make-believe hospital where toys were being treated for various ailments. I didn't have to do anything; I was the nurse, a live prop. She loved pretending she was the doctor, bossing me around, being in charge. Because she was making it up as she went along, she enjoyed 'knowing' more than me about what we were doing. Easy!

2. Watch your child do something (Age 1+) My daughter has always loved to have me watch her play. She is an only child (in my house); maybe it's just the company she enjoys but it may be more than that. I think it's important to her that I see what she is doing and she can share it with me, even if I'm not directly involved in the activity. It can be "Watch me dance, Mum!" or "Can you watch my concert?" Not every child demands an audience. I think all children like to feel that what they are doing is worth watching. They, like everyone, love to feel valued! It's a way for them to confirm in their minds that "You see me," "I am worthy of your attention" and "I'm important to you."

The key to creating quality time is to stay present and absorb the beauty of watching your child play. Enjoy observing their movements, their imagination, their commentary. The key is not to let your mind drift to other things!

3. Watch 10 minutes of their favourite show with them (Age 3+) We have a reward system with my daughter. I told her once that for her particularly good behaviour in a not-so-easy situation, she'd get a reward that evening. She said, "Can you watch one of my shows, Mum?" Kids love it when you do kid things with them; it's important for building stronger bonds. Many episodes of television shows for young kids only play for about 10 minutes. Of course, I subtly guide her to watch something that doesn't drive me crazy, but for 10-15 minutes I can put up with anything. She thinks I'm wonderful for doing so!

4. Play cards (Age 3+) At a young age, kids can follow simple card games like Snap, Go Fish and Uno. If you don't get too hung up on rules, cards can be fun for both the kids and parents. When little kids naively show their hand of cards and ask, "Do I have a Jack, Mum?" the temptation is to tell them not to show your cards. They have no attachments to winning or losing; they're just in it for fun. We parents can learn from that! The beauty of playing cards is that you can do it with older children, too, and it's easy to do while lying in bed!

5. Play a Board Game (Age 3+) Depending on the game, most kids from about age 3 can play board games or manual games. Connect 4 is an easy one to start with then you can graduate to harder ones such as Othello, Mastermind, Scrabble, all the way up to Monopoly.

For chronically ill parents, simpler games that don't need much space or brain power are probably best. Othello, Mastermind and Connect 4 fit the bill here and the first two are great for older kids, as well. Most of these games can be played in multiple sessions over multiple days which helps when you don't have much energy or brain power available. They can also be played while lying in bed.

Have fun!

How I Maintain A Social Life With Chronic Illness
By Mary Pettigrew

Maintaining a social life when you have a chronic illness can be challenging. There are times when I can make plans and follow through with friends and family but often I cancel, sometimes at the last minute. The fatigue factor and the unpredictable nature of multiple sclerosis (MS) are most often the reasons for cancelled plans or complete avoidance of making plans at all.

Changing my plans is most frustrating to my mother but she's getting better at dealing with it as the years go by. She tells me I've become "predictably unpredictable." My friends get disappointed but they truly love me and always understand. Unless it's an early dinner with my mother, I no longer go out in the evening. I do not drive after dark unless it's in my neighborhood. I prefer to meet people for breakfast or lunch. I'm getting much better at explaining why without feeling guilty or "weird" for my limitations. I'm lucky to have the friends with whom I grew up, as well as new friends I've met online and through participation in MS fundraisers.

It's been years since I've dated. If someone attempts to get flirty with me within my online circles, I shut that down immediately. I tried dating a few times after my divorce, met a few nice guys who seemed unfazed by my MS but a second date never came to be. In fact, some never called or texted after that. I also realized I was quite damaged from my divorce and other issues with my ex-husband so I decided to seek out a psychiatrist. I found a doctor who fit me incredibly well and I still see her to this day. I have also chosen to remain celibate with no plans or desire to change my status. This choice may not be right for others, but it is right for me.

I have a large community of friends and acquaintances online. I engage with them often, interacting with people who have a variety of interests such as MS, chronic illness, music, poetry, writing, blogging and film/theater. Many of the friends I've met via Twitter and Facebook have become true friends! We sometimes get together or at least chat on the phone when we can. In fact, I met Carolyn on Twitter. She has MS and was living in California when we met. Eventually she and her husband moved here to Texas and now live only 45 minutes away! We've become best friends...soul sisters.

I tell people, "I live alone but I'm not lonely" and this is true. I have a dog and a cat – my companions who give me unconditional love. When I'm having bad days or weeks, I tend to hunker down with my TV. When I don't have the energy or focus to write, I use note pads and Post-It notes to jot down ideas, thoughts or interesting quotes I come across. The creative juices eventually return and it's great to have a little stack of idea prompts to play with.

Writing is my passion – especially poetry. Expressing myself in this manner has become my best therapy. I generally write for myself but the bonus comes when someone reads my work and connects to it emotionally. That's a WOW! I enjoy other forms of creative writing but poetry works well for me because it's a short burst of emotion via words. I can compose several poems in one sitting then move on to the next project or topic.

I'm filled with passion but I do tend to take on too many projects. My brain can only focus for so long, my vision gets blurry and eventually I'm swimming in a sea of paper and unfinished projects. It is what it is. I'm me and although I frustrate myself and others at times, I wouldn't change things for the world. It's all good.

Survival At The Grocery Store And In The Kitchen
By Melanie Styles

What stresses me most is grocery shopping with a migraine and fibro fog: I get the grocery store equivalent of road rage. I learned to survive teaching in a classroom during my worst health crises by planning ahead and following through, step-by-step. To help conserve my energy and time, and lessen my stress, I decided to apply those techniques to grocery shopping, organizing my kitchen and other aspects of life with chronic illness.

Let's plan a successful grocery-shopping trip together!

- <u>Rest</u>: You increase your chances of having an incident-free shopping trip if you are well-rested.
- <u>Eat</u>: Eat something before you go. Experts tell you to do this to avoid buying junk. I want you to eat because a dip in blood sugar can make you angry or irritable. Pain and anger are an ugly mix; you don't want to end up on a wanted poster!
- <u>Plan</u>: If shopping has been a problem in the past, get a map of your favorite store and use it to plan your trips. Snap pictures in the store so that you know what is featured in each aisle. As you look at the map and your pictures, organize your list according to your route through the store. I use coupons, so I put the coupons in this order, too. I also mark my list with a little symbol that reminds me to match that item to the coupon, as it may require a certain size or amount.

Now you are ready to go to the store.

- <u>Buddy up</u>: Whether you live alone or not, find a shopping buddy. I recommend finding someone to help you unpack the groceries, as well. If you can only get one or the other, which is more helpful to you?
- <u>Loading the cart</u>: Put groceries into the cart in an order that makes sense to you. You can organize by:
  - Budget- Separate items you may not be able to afford in one spot in your cart and ones you know you can afford in another;

- o Pricing- When I am price matching, I separate those items from regular priced items in my cart so I can get the cashier to change the prices.
- Organization- I place groceries onto the belt the way I want them bagged together. It takes a little time but it helps me put them away more quickly.
- Bagging: Don't forget to ask your checker or bagger to bag the groceries lightly.
- Unloading: Consider having someone else load and unload the car or use a wagon to pull the bags into the house.
- Unpacking: When you get home, put the bags down where most of the contents belong: near the pantry or fridge, in the bathroom. I put refrigerated items away while helpers unload the car, then take a break before I organize the rest of the groceries.
- Order online: I used to walk around shops for hours. Now I order as much as I can online to be delivered to my home, or at the very least order ahead to have it waiting at the store for pickup. Can you do that with prescriptions? Toilet paper? Groceries?

Kitchen Organization for Ease

The way that you organize your kitchen is personal and depends on your lifestyle, but it can also make a big difference in your energy use and motivation to cook or clean. I found I can fit more food in my refrigerator and see its contents better by adding clear refrigerator organizers on the shelves and encourage my family to keep the food organized in them. I have a special diet so I keep my foods and healthy snacks in a particular place where I can grab them quickly and easily.

We have a deep freeze. I tend to drop things because of my illness so I put food groups into canvas bags that I can pick up by the handles and pull out of the freezer, instead of fishing through the freezer item by item.

In the pantry, refrigerator and freezer you can find what you're looking for more easily if you store by category:

Meal – For example, everything you need to make lasagna, a sandwich, or tacos
Time of day - Breakfast, Lunch, Snacks and Dinner
Food Group – Meats, Breads, Dairy, Vegetables

Easy Self-Care
By Cameron Auxer

Whether you have been ill for years or for a few days, had surgery, injury or an emotional upset, there are times when we want a mommy. But, alas, we are grownups; we must take care of ourselves. Taking care of our bodies and minds is important even when we are well. It becomes vital when we are not. When we are experiencing physical or emotional pain we must give ourselves a hug, create a positive inner dialogue, nourish our bodies and souls, and soothe our discomfort.

Here are some easy ways to give yourself some Tender Loving Care (Note: these recommendations should not replace professional medical care or therapy):

Rest. Whether you nap, wrap yourself in a blanket with a cup of cocoa and a good book, or binge-watch Netflix, give your body some quality rest. If you aren't sleeping well at night, dim the lights and try a warm Epsom salt bath with a few drops of lavender oil, accompanied by your favorite relaxing music. Do this before bedtime and try to go to bed at the same time each night. Stay off electronic devices within an hour of going to bed, and if your device allows, turn off the blue light.

Snip some posies from your garden. Even a tiny bouquet of violets in a glass can lift your spirits. Or have someone fetch a cheap bouquet from a local store. The lovely color and fragrance of flowers will lift the energy in your room, as well as your spirits.

Cuddle furbabies. The purr of a cat can lower your stress and blood pressure. Pets of any kind can help improve your emotional and physical health. Their unconditional love is a bonus. If you can't keep a pet, have a friend bring their furbaby for a visit. If you are allergic to animals, cuddle a stuffed animal. Either way, you will feel comforted.

Dim the lights. Twist your dimmer switch or light a candle. If you can tolerate scented candles, buy those that have a nostalgic scent that floods you with good memories. If you are sensitive to scents, use unscented candles or LED candles if you want to avoid open flames. Scented or unscented, go with ones made from beeswax or organic palm oil that have no lead in the wicks. Instant relaxation!

Say Ohm or Amen. Whether you pray or meditate, you transport yourself to a higher place beyond your pain. Even if you just take just 5 minutes a day to pay attention to your breathing or pray you can lower your blood pressure, ease stress and clear your head. Guided meditation cds can be very helpful if you have a "monkey mind."

Take a dose of Music Medicine. More and more research touts the benefits of music to help alleviate pain and stress, lower blood pressure and generally support your well-being. To relax deeply, sacred music or soft instrumentals will transport you to a restful state. You can lift your spirits and your energy with your favorite rock (Motown does it for me). With so many online music services these days you can easily stream or download your favorite tunes to create your own special mixes to suit your mood.

Inspire yourself! There are myriad books, magazines, cds, tv shows, films, websites and YouTube channels that offer all sorts of inspiring material to improve your well-being and help you to think more positively. Sometimes all you need is a little change in perspective to get through a tough time.

Eat real food. Comfort food does not have to be unhealthy. A warm bowl of oatmeal…macaroni and cheese…mashed potatoes…yummy soup – all these things can be made from healthy ingredients. If the list of ingredients is a mile long, contains unpronounceable chemicals and has been dead or removed from the earth for a long, long time, it's better laid to rest in the garbage can. Eat freshly made foods (organic, if possible) or at least healthy organic brands of prepared convenience foods. Drink fresh juices as opposed to pasteurized bottled juice. Google "anti-inflammatory foods" and follow the recommendations. And above all, eat your fruits and veggies! Your body depends on good fuel to maintain and to heal itself. The quality of food you eat is similar to the octane level of gasoline for your car. The higher the quality, the better your engine will run!

Your nose knows. Aromatherapy using essential oils is a most enjoyable, indulgent way to care for yourself. You can use these aromatic oils in a diffuser or add them to your bath or body products. Find websites that educate you on which oils will help your special needs. For example, lavender is calming, peppermint is uplifting. Rosemary is good for brain fog. Be sure to check for sensitivities or allergy warnings if you use aromatherapy oils on your skin and don't overdo the amount of oil used in your diffuser. Usually 1 drop in water is enough.

Bodywork works. There are many types of bodywork to help ease pain and provide relaxation. It's important to find a style that feels good to you and is helpful with what ails you. Even more important is to find practitioners who are certified and get good reviews or references. Always, always, always talk with a practitioner before you get bodywork to discuss your chronic condition. There are many types of massage and there is a plethora of therapies available such as craniosacral therapy, reflexology, Shiatsu and acupuncture that can help with symptoms. I prefer Reiki which is a safe, passive, relaxing method that gently transfers healing energy into your body through the hands. Read books, research online and ask your friends for their experiences with bodywork. Find the modality and experienced practitioner that is right for you.

Give a hug, get a hug. Hugging is the best therapy in the world! Hug a friend, hug your loved one, hug a pet. If there is no one in reach, hug a stuffed animal or a hot water bottle. Hugs are good medicine – research says so!

LOL. You can exercise your internal organs, flood your body with good chemicals and temporarily forget your pain when you have a good hearty laugh. Watch funny movies and tv shows. Listen to old radio comedy and recordings of stand-up comedians. Read humorous books. With a good sense of humor, you'll find reasons to laugh everywhere!

Visit your Mother Nature. A short leisurely walk in nature is invigorating; it clears the mind and fills the lungs with fresh air. If you are unable to walk, sit outside and let your senses absorb that beautiful day. When bedbound, ask someone to open windows, set out flowers, or pop in a cd with nature sounds. Let Mother Nature lift your spirits daily!

Just because it's natural, doesn't mean it isn't toxic. Someone may tell you that an herbal supplement worked like magic for their condition and there are lots of ads that promise miracle cures. Please be smart and only take herbal supplements with the guidance of a qualified practitioner. Though some formulas can be effective for certain conditions, the dosage, strength and side effects may vary and toxic interactions may occur when taken with certain medications or foods. Herbs can be powerful so be cautious and wise.

Say NO! One of the best things you can do for yourself is set firm boundaries with others, especially if you have been a people-pleaser most of your life. We enjoy being independent but when we are ill, it's time to ask of others instead of harming your health by trying to serve their every need.

When you take good care of yourself, you raise your quality of life and your general well-being. Sometimes with chronic illness, especially where there is no cure, that's the best we can ask for!

Travelling With Chronic Illness
By Siân Wootton

When you're diagnosed with a chronic illness your world changes. Getting out of bed is a challenge, let alone leaving the house. I'm fortunate enough to have travelled since my diagnosis and becoming a wheelchair user so I'd like to share some things I've learned to make travelling as a chronically ill person more achievable for you.

Be honest with yourself and realistic about your abilities; what kind of travel can you manage, how far can you travel and for how long? Exhausting yourself from the travel then being too unwell for the duration of your stay defeats the purpose. Be honest about with whom you can travel. Having an understanding caregiver who is happy to move at your pace is very different from travelling with friends who want action-packed adventure leaving you all alone.

Research is essential to find a destination and accommodation that meets your needs. List the desired characteristics of a destination and available facilities that you require to narrow your search. Find as much information as needed to make a choice that is right for you. TripAdvisor reviews, forums and photos online are helpful, as well as talking to facilities' management directly. If you want wheelchair accessible accommodation, research what that means for each place and look carefully at photos. Unfortunately, the meaning of "accessible" can vary significantly and different standards apply in different countries. Knowledge can help reduce anxiety. Your destination and accommodation need to feel like a new comfort zone.

When booking travel insurance always declare your condition(s) and any hospital stays within the past year. Failing to do so can render your insurance invalid. Unless you are at significant risk there is often no extra expense. You may also wish to consider a policy that covers your medical equipment.

Whether you're a regular wheelchair user or have reduced mobility, booking special assistance makes tackling the madness in airports much easier. You can book assistance online but it's best to call your airline's special assistance line to see what's offered to meet your needs and ensure that it's available for your flight. The airline is responsible for booking services at both your departure and arrival airports, as well as on-board. They can advise you on the medical equipment you can take with you free-of-charge, in addition to your luggage allowance and the safety requirements for power chairs and scooters. You can also pre-book appropriate seats. Ask questions about where you need to go in the airport to register and check-in, as each airport is different. You can also find this information on the airport's website.

Order medication for your trip well in advance with enough to cover any delays or extra dosages you may need, such as pain killers for flares. Also have enough meds for the week after your holiday, in case you are too unwell to reorder or get to the pharmacy once you get home. Check airline guidelines on liquid medications (especially if you exceed the 3oz liquid limit for carry-on luggage), syringes or medication that needs refrigeration. Pack them all in your hand luggage so they will not go missing in lost checked baggage, in their original labelled packaging, along with a doctor's letter or written prescription with your name and address, for customs and security purposes.

Speaking of packing, make detailed lists that you or someone packing on your behalf can easily follow. It may benefit you to bring a brief medical history, medication list with dosages and amount you take daily, allergy list, physician name and contact information, next of kin information, health insurance information and anything else pertinent should you need medical treatment while abroad. You may also want to include power-of-attorney paperwork or your living will if you feel it is necessary. These may be helpful in the case of hospitalization should you become seriously ill and unable to speak for yourself.

Bear in mind the climate you're going to, the activities you intend to do and the length of your stay. Pack everything that you'd need on your worst day; for me that means taking an electric heat pad to Greece. It's always best to be over-prepared.

Pack essentials in your hand luggage (mindful of any regulations) to help in case of a flare during the journey. Within my hand luggage I carry a "grab bag" - a small clutch bag which I keep on my seat beside me for quick access to items I may need. Mainly I pack travel bands (for air or sea sickness), medication for during the flight, straws for drinks, face wipes and lavender roll-on. This means I don't have to rummage through my main hand luggage, especially if I'm feeling sick or dizzy during take-off, landing or the dreaded turbulence.

Airports and planes can be noisy and uncomfortable. Pack headphones, travel pillows and a sleep mask. Dress comfortably with shoes you can easily slip off and an extra pair of socks to avoid cold feet. A large scarf can double as a blanket. Sunglasses can help headaches and dizziness from the sun's glare. Compression stockings help restless or sore legs and reduce swelling (*Editor's note: They also prevent dangerous deep-vein thrombosis*). If the plane is not full, ask for a row to yourself to be able to sit with your legs up or if your travel companions don't mind put your legs across them. If you have a long flight, make sure you try to get up and let some blood circulate every hour or so. If you can walk to the bathroom then do so, but if you cannot, try to stand at your seat and shake your legs a bit.

Whilst you're away, be mindful that you will still get symptoms and need a lot of rest. Listen to your body and go at your own pace. Keeping a routine bed time can be helpful. Try to avoid sunburn. Be careful with what you eat if you have allergies or intolerances. www.celiactravel.com is a great resource for eating in foreign countries with food allergies. Don't forget to drink plenty of bottled water as travelling can be very dehydrating. Beware of tap water while traveling. The last thing you want is a GI upset to ruin your trip!

Understandably, you may be apprehensive before setting off. Be grateful for this new adventure. Most importantly, give yourself a pat on the back and go forth to enjoy the experience as much as you can. You are brave, bold, courageous and no illness will prevent you from living life to the fullest. Go out there and see the world!

For in-depth information and travel interviews, please visit www.howtodealwithme.blogspot.com.

Chapter 4
Becoming Your Own Best Health Care Advocate

Advocating For Yourself With Your Doctors
By Dennis Maione

I am my own best advocate. What about all those who know better than I do? The professionals who understand disease and healing? Who am I to question their treatment plan or, heaven forbid, bring forward my own ideas?

When it comes to how you feel, no one knows better than you. You might not be able to label organs or glands on a diagram, but you know your body. You know when you're sick and when you're in pain. You may not be able to tell the difference between pain caused by your body and that caused by your mind but both are real and need to be dealt with.

If you have a chronic illness, you've been through drugs and therapies. You've seen your symptoms come and go and you know when certain things work and when they don't. You know you. As a result, you've got a lot to offer your medical team.

Sometimes, like me, your condition is rare enough that you're one of the experts. Sometimes, like me, you have enough uneasiness when faced with a treatment plan that you want a second opinion: expert help in choosing a treatment that makes sense to you, with consequences you can live with.

Let's talk a bit about advocating for yourself.

What Does Self-Advocacy Look Like?

Sometimes it seems self-advocacy is a big deal, involving conflict, demands and third-party assistance. Sometimes it feels like shouting at the top of your lungs or holding your breath until you're blue. Usually it's nothing you haven't done before: asking about what's happening to you. Clarifying the reasoning, timing and implications of treatment. Asking about options until you're satisfied about the best course of action. Sometimes it's the simple statement: "I'd like a second opinion."

When Should I Self-Advocate?

Since self-advocacy can be as simple as learning about what's going to happen to you, the answer to "When should I self-advocate?" is easy:

always! While that's true, certain circumstances are red flags telling you to go out of your way to find out more and perhaps choose a new direction. The list below (not complete) signals instances when to take special care to put the brakes on:

1. When you don't understand what's going to be done.

You need to understand your treatment. Is there going to be a surgery or other invasive procedure? Drug therapies? If your doctor won't or can't explain the planned treatments in a way that you can understand AND to your satisfaction, it's time to ask more questions. If you still can't get satisfaction from the doctor, ask someone else. In the end, unless you fully understand what and why, never proceed with a treatment. Never let a doctor do something to you simply because he or she says it's best.

2. When the probable result isn't something you're willing to live with.

Do you know what the possible results of your treatment are? If you're told that a procedure has an 80% chance of leaving you unable to speak, you need to ask whether you're willing to live with that result. If not, you need to ask what other options are available.

It's possible there is no best probable outcome. Being thoroughly educated about the options, however, will help you make the best decision for you. You can't afford to assume you'll be the one long-shot to get that best outcome. Having wrestled with the reality that a difficult treatment may not extend your life with the quality you require, you need to determine whether you truly want that treatment or not.

3. When your medical team isn't considering important facts about you, your body or your circumstances. Or they are NOT listening to you!

Not everyone with condition 'X' is the same: if something in your genetics, history or environment is not typical, your presentation or treatment of condition 'X' might be different as well. If you know something unique about yourself that's not being taken into consideration start a conversation with your doctor. If they are not hearing you, keep repeating until they actually LISTEN.

The second time I got cancer, I knew I had Lynch syndrome, a genetic condition that creates tumours with different molecular structures. My

139

oncologist insisted on treating me as a standard colon cancer patient, even after I presented articles from reputable medical journals that called his treatment into question. Try as I might, I couldn't get him to discuss the evidence I'd found. I went to great lengths to get an informed second opinion—one which took my genetics into consideration. It reversed the first opinion and I made an informed choice.

4. When the process is going too fast or too slow.

Someone said, "Timing is everything," and that's especially true in medicine. Too often, we find ourselves concerned about how long it's taking to see a doctor, get a diagnosis or test result, or begin treatment. Sometimes these delays can result in dangerous disease progression.

On the other hand, speed is sometimes the villain; eagerness to get your treatment underway can blind your medical team to other options. Mostly every situation benefits from patience and due time for careful assessment.

5. When you're uncomfortable with anything in the diagnosis or treatment process.

This is a catch-all for anything about which you feel uncomfortable. It may be the treatment facility is too far away from your family, the primary doctor gives you an odd feeling, or the pills are just too large! Even if you're worried your concern may not seem reasonable, you have the right to talk it over, have all your questions answered and be comfortable with what's going to happen. Never forget that the doctor may have a degree but he/she is just a person like you who is there to help you. Do not fear them or make decisions because they put any pressure on you. Follow your instincts. If it doesn't feel right, it isn't right.

Advocating for yourself will sometimes be hard. Medical professionals may be confused as to why you're speaking up or angry because they feel you've invaded their domain. That's okay. You are not there to become their friends. You are seeking the best treatment for YOUR body and that is the bottom line. Better to be thought a disruptive person than let others have undue control over your health and destiny.

Help Others To Help You
By Elizabeth Turp

When we are diagnosed with a chronic condition, especially if uncommon, we need assistance – physically, emotionally, in and out of the house and navigating the health care system. You must learn to help others so that they can help you.

First, you must help yourself:

Accept where you are

While it can be a relief to get a diagnosis, it's natural to resist the thought of lifelong difficulties that come with it. You may try to continue with life as it was, pushing beyond your limits. The best thing you can do is listen to your body and find ways to adapt. You may think that means giving in to ill health but it's actually the opposite. Listening to your body can be the most important thing you do to help yourself and help others help you. Overdoing it uses precious energy, increases stress and can make symptoms worse. Accept you are ill and improve your quality of life.

Make self-management your priority

Your most important job now is to manage your illness. If this is difficult because you also care for others, know you will be better able to look after them if you look after yourself. There are many things you can do: nutrition, movement, relaxation, emotional support, massage, meditation and physiotherapy. What do others say works for them? Be wary of anything expensive or promising a cure and remember that not doing self-care can lead to worsening of your condition.

Understand the mind-body connection

Western medicine and culture tend to split the body into parts and separate mental and physical health. The reality is that long-term physical illness impacts mental health through isolation, anxiety, frustration, depression, anger, grief, guilt and shame. Emotional difficulties can also negatively impact physical symptoms and coping, making self-care harder and pain, fatigue and brain fog worse. You can't afford to ignore this - being open to holistic self-care and seeking emotional support are key to living well with chronic illness.

Focus on what you can do

You are not your illness; you are a person who has an illness. Acknowledge what it takes to get you through the day. People with chronic conditions can be equal in determination, focus and courage to Olympic athletes! Keep space in your life for interests and pleasures. Be careful with whom you engage. Some online communities and real-life support groups can be negative, focusing on searching for cures and injustice. While these are real issues, they are not the best way to spend limited energy. Find support that helps develop positive coping strategies, decreasing stress and inflammation.

Now help others help you:

Find good explanations of your condition(s) and pass them on

Have a simple description of your illness to give out so people know what you're facing. Whether it's a book, blog, article, leaflet, patient.info or Christine Miserandino's 'Spoon Theory,' find something to put into words about your complex experience. Offer the information, suggesting that reading it will help them help you. I wrote my book for this very reason.

Be assertive

Asking for help after being independent can be challenging but is vital. If you don't voice your needs, they won't be met. Healthcare professionals are often pressed for time and may lack empathic skills required to tease information out of you. Take a trusted person with you to appointments. Ask them to help prepare what you want to say beforehand, make your points while you're there and, afterwards, they can help you remember what was said by taking notes during the visit. This helps if you have brain fog and ensures opportunities aren't missed. Honesty about symptoms and concerns is crucial; you know yourself best and deserve individualised support.

Address any barriers to asking for help

Illness brings great change. Especially with invisible conditions, others may not understand the changes and their usual expectations of you may continue. You need to explain. You may find it difficult changing from a 'helper' role to the one who needs help. You may also experience guilt, feeling that you can't 'bother' others for help. Turn guilt on its head with the idea that to continue to be someone who cares about others, you must take care of yourself first. If you are stuck in shame or can't accept your situation, counselling may help.

Use the law: it's your right to get what you need

Equality and disability laws are there to protect and assist you. Unfortunately, organisations don't always put these into practice, so familiarise yourself with what applies to you. For example, in the UK, The Equality Act (2010) makes it a legal requirement for employers to make 'reasonable adjustments' to the role of someone with a disabling illness so they can do their job. Seek out union reps, charity helplines, benefits and disability rights advisors to help others support you to get what you need.

Get real about your support systems

One of the hardest things about chronic illness is how it changes relationships. With people who ignore, deny or minimise your illness, pull back - don't waste energy on those who don't try to understand. Be aware of how you come across: you may be telling others how ill you are but also how well you cope. People tend to hear the positive and miss the suffering underneath. If you 'look fine' the brutal truth about your illness is key, at least with people close to you. You may find the support you need in unexpected places. Things have changed for you but it's not all bad. Taking control of your own care can lead to reduced symptoms, better support and a deep appreciation for the simple things in life.

Getting Care When You're Rural
By Erica Rogers

I look out of the bay window in my kitchen and I can see forever. On a calm winter morning, I swear I can see the sun reflecting off the east face of the Rocky Mountains in Colorado. It's quiet, it's beautiful and it brings me peace. I chose to live in a rural area. To me, this is perfect.

There are advantages to living in a "fly-over state." Small communities are scattered every 30 miles or so. Not many people "travel to" rural Northwestern Kansas. If you come here you're visiting family or moving here. From the front porch, I can watch the planes fly back and forth from Denver International Airport and I'm sure as they look down on the patchwork of corn fields they ask themselves, "Why would someone live there?" But I love it!

Living in a rural area does have its challenges. You must plan your trips to town accordingly; you can't forget anything or you'll have to make the 45-mile round trip again. As winter weather approaches, you mentally run through the checklist of things that need to be done. Planning becomes an art form and you learn to do it with perfection.

What happens when things aren't planned? There is no medical "weatherman" to warn me of impending health challenges. I can't just "stock up" on drugs for multiple sclerosis or pop in for an MRI next time I am in town.

When my local urgent care clinic (local means 2 hours away) suggested that I see a neurologist, I knew that I would face challenges. I turned to the internet and searched for "neurologists near me" which equaled: no results found. I knew that I had two choices...Denver, Colorado (3.5 hours away) or Wichita, Kansas (5 hours away). I spent the next 2 hours searching for a doctor that had good credentials and could see me soon. I found a center in Denver that could see me in two days.

Find the doctor – done! I had to coordinate the trip. How early did I have to leave to make it there in plenty of time? How bad would the traffic be? How long does it take to get downtown? What is the weather report? Is it going to snow that day?

I made the fateful 3.5-hour journey to Denver and met my doctor for the first of many visits. Then I made the 3.5-hour trip home with many things heavy on my mind and heart. There's quiet solitude in driving for miles down a desolate road, only passing a car every 30 miles. Having to travel to and from the doctor at this distance gives you time to think.

The months to follow were cluttered with carefully planned MRIs, return visits to the neurologist and medical tests that had to be done in Denver because no one local had the equipment. I now have the path to and from my doctor's office memorized. I also learned that 10 miles in Northwestern Kansas is NOT the same as 10 miles in Denver, Colorado. I never imagined it would take 45 minutes to go 10 miles in a city!

Preparation is key, yet things still happen that mess up a well-thought-out plan. In November, I had an appointment at 1:45pm and planned to leave home at 9am to give me plenty of time to get there. As I got ready that morning, I looked outside. Overnight it had snowed 10 inches. There was a 4-foot snow drift in front of my garage door. That appointment had to be rescheduled.

There are many wonderful things about living in rural America and I wouldn't trade it for anything in the world. Just as it is important for you to prepare for bad weather, it is equally important that you advocate for your health. If you don't agree or don't feel comfortable with the local medical professional's opinion, seek advice elsewhere. Don't be afraid to travel outside of your comfort zone, find a specialist and keep looking until you are confident that you have found the right one.

Call your insurance company and determine what steps will be necessary to cover an out-of-state doctor's visit. In my case, it was a simple matter but make sure you have referrals if needed. Make use of your support system; lean on family and friends, find a travel partner and plan on overnight trips if you can't travel for long periods of time. Schedule several appointments together if you can. Have tests run in the morning and see the doctor in the afternoon. Always take an overnight bag, including your medicine, in case something comes up and you must stay.

Explore the resources available for travel expense assistance. You may find assistance at the county or state level but you should also consider organizations like the National Patient Travel Center (www.patienttravel.org), Patient Airlift Services (www.palservices.org) and Mercy Medical Airlift (www.mercymedical.org). Additionally, Amtrak gives disability discounts. Don't forget to reach out to support groups because people may be willing to open their home to you for a night if you need to stay. Some large hospitals also have discounts at hotel rooms for patients.

Above all, don't regret your decision to live in a rural area because you need to travel for medical treatment. Find comfort in the peace your home brings you. Take advantage of the tranquil nights and the calm mornings. Find joy in living in a "fly-over state." Being happy at home may be the best thing you ever do for your health.

When You're Not Visibly Disabled
By Suzanne Robins

If you were to meet me today you'd think there was nothing wrong with me. Though I've been living with multiple sclerosis (MS) for more than 20 years, I'm not visibly disabled in any way. One side of my face is numb, I've lost the grip in my writing hand and my left foot drops a bit when I walk. But I don't need a cane, crutches or a wheelchair; in terms of physical mobility, I'm doing very well.

I know I'm one of the fortunate ones and I thank my lucky stars every day for what I'm still capable of doing. I am walking without support, sitting down and standing up, climbing stairs, speaking clearly, grasping things, feeding myself, going to the bathroom on my own and driving anywhere I want to go. Over the years, I've experienced a range of invisible MS symptoms - including depression, anxiety, bladder dysfunction, cognitive impairment and fatigue – all of which have crippled my life in other ways. They've stolen my confidence, eroded my strengths and battered my self-esteem.

Getting others to appreciate and understand the hidden impact of my illness has been my greatest challenge. When there's no cane or wheelchair to signal disability, people assume it isn't there. When I share how I'm doing, I sometimes feel like my friends and family think that I'm exaggerating my symptoms or making them up. Most people are too polite to say it but the disbelief is written on their faces. How can you possibly be feeling so bad, when you're looking so good?

I've found this skepticism extends to my physicians as well. Even my neurologist seems doubtful at times and who could blame him? My symptoms are mild compared to those of many other patients. His assessment of how I'm doing and my description of how I'm feeling are often vastly different. Even doctors tend to assume that all is well, when everything appears to be fine. Looks can be deceiving.

This explains, in part, why it took almost a decade for me to get a diagnosis. Though I'd complained for years about chronic insomnia and bladder problems, I could never get my family physician to take me seriously. No matter what issue I came to her with, it was always dismissed. I was in and out of her office so many times, I wondered if she thought I was a hypochondriac.

When I was finally diagnosed with MS, I was furious with her for having missed it. The clues were all there and she'd failed to connect the dots. I railed at her incompetence and blamed her for allowing my problems to spiral out of control for so long.

I was mad at myself, as well, for not pushing harder for answers to my medical concerns. I had let her off the hook too easily and allowed her to dismiss my complaints. I should have pressed her for more testing. I should have insisted on seeing a specialist sooner. I should have found another doctor when I was dissatisfied with her care.

That was on me. I promised myself I would never let it happen again.

Since then, I've been much more aggressive - and persistent - in advocating on my own behalf. When new symptoms emerged several years later, I refused to let it go. I was having problems with dizziness, extreme fatigue, swollen joints, numbness in my fingers and toes, and a high resting heart rate. I couldn't get my doctor to look past my MS and consider other causes.

This time I kept pushing for answers until blood tests finally revealed that I had an iron deficiency. Once that was corrected, all the symptoms I was experiencing disappeared. Finally, I had an explanation for why I'd been feeling so rotten and it wasn't my MS, as my doctor had automatically assumed.

That was enough to convince me to find another primary care physician; one who listens attentively, answers all my questions patiently and doesn't dismiss my concerns. Securing the medical treatment I need is now a straightforward process. I no longer feel like I'm begging to be heard or like I'm the one who's "steering the bus."

That doesn't mean that I've taken my foot off the pedal. My experience has taught me I must be the driving force behind my care. I can't sit back and hope that I'll get answers. I must keep asking questions until I do.

I was reminded of that recently when a routine MRI raised questions about my original diagnosis. Though my neurologist was confident that he'd made the right call, I immediately pressed for a second opinion - even though I knew it might compromise our relationship. It scared me to think that I might have been injecting myself with a powerful drug for the wrong illness all this time and I needed to know for certain that I was treating the right thing.

The other specialist started from scratch and reassessed everything by taking a detailed medical history, reviewing my chart, performing her own neurological exam and ordering more tests. In the end, she came to the same conclusion as my own neurologist: I have MS. It wasn't a wasted effort. Having my case reexamined by a second set of eyes has given me tremendous peace of mind and renewed confidence that I'm receiving the appropriate care.

Portions of this article are taken from my book "Faulty Wiring: Living with Invisible MS."

The Take-Charge Patient's Toolkit
By Martine Ehrenclou, M.A.

Taking charge of YOU as a patient is essential in today's complex health care system. The more informed you are about all aspects of your medical care, the more the quality of care you receive will improve. If you actively participate in your care, you will experience better care, increased patient safety, increased patient satisfaction and more. This is about becoming your own best advocate.

The Take-Charge Patient's Toolkit found in the Appendix contains questions, checklists and forms to help you become a take-charge patient, so you can feel more confidence and be in control. By inserting your information into the Health Summary, Health History and Medical ID Card, and preparing questions before your medical appointments, you'll not only converse with your doctors more confidently but you'll prevent medical errors, as well.

Use the forms, questions and checklists as companion pieces with my book, The Take-Charge Patient, or simply as quick-and-easy aids. Copy and fill them out before your next medical appointment either with your current medical provider or a new doctor or specialist. Take these with you and check the forms as your office visit proceeds.

Note: Forms, questions and checklists can be found in Appendix

Chapter 5
Your Passion, Your Purpose and Starting Over

Rising From The Ashes

You've been diagnosed with a chronic illness and it feels like your life as you knew it has ended. You will grieve for the life you had; you NEED to grieve as part of your healing process. After you pick yourself up and dust yourself off, you may start to wonder what to do with the rest of your life. Time to identify what your passion is – what rings your bell, inspires you, brings you joy, what you're good at and what you are still able to do. This is something about which you shouldn't have to think too hard. Passion bubbles under the surface, even while being ignored.

Finding your passion leads to discovering your purpose for this time in life. Purpose gives your life meaning. It creates opportunity to contribute to others, feed your passion and nourish your soul. You may have always had a strong sense of purpose or a current career path; to continue in that direction will require flexibility and adjustment to your new limitations. This isn't Mission Impossible. Where there is a will, there is a way.

If you had felt that your life was lacking purpose before you became ill or if you had been dissatisfied with the direction your life was taking, then this is the PERFECT opportunity to create something BRAND NEW!

You don't have to go out and save the world. You don't have to make earth-shaking and paradigm-shattering discoveries or inventions. Your purpose can range from writing a blog or creating lovely things for others to enjoy, to establishing a foundation to raise awareness for your disease. Even making phone calls for a cause is a vital contribution. Technology gives us the ability to connect with others and avoid isolation, as well as conduct business and earn income from our home.

This chapter assists you in finding your passion and purpose and creating a new life. Just like a young bird, your wings may be weak and shaky; you may feel vulnerable and insecure. Remember, you are now officially, a Chronic Illness Warrior and you're about to take flight into a new life. Our wish for you is that you SOAR!

Starting Over
By Anne Gaucher
Aka "Lyme Lens"

I never understood the desperation of unemployment until it was thrust upon me. I got my first job at fourteen at a corner grocery store. Throughout my life, I've always held a job. It would be foreign to me not to collect a paycheck, even though there have been times that I despised what I was doing.

Before I got sick, I enjoyed rewarding careers of service to others. I was blessed to find my calling in life. I sacrificed a lot to have a career; it was a huge priority. That came to a screeching halt in 2011.

Maybe you experienced something similar. One day you're doing your job, collecting a paycheck, utilizing skills you spent a decade perfecting, when suddenly you're stricken with an illness and can no longer work. Everything gone in an instant and it's completely out of your control.

Some people say, "Hallelujah! I hated that job. I can finally lie on the couch and get caught up on my rest!" That feeling lasts about two weeks, then panic sets in when the paychecks stop but the bills keep coming. The frenzy to find employment begins as you realize that you're not prepared for the loss. You grapple with the facts that you're too sick to work, your benefits only last so long, you now have enormous medical bills compounding the financial crisis and you have no idea when you'll be well enough work...if ever. Reality has begun to set in.

Other people who loved their job may say, "I'm devastated! How could this be happening? Not only am I sick but I've also lost a major part of who I AM. That job was important to me! I made a difference and now I've lost that, too. A huge piece of my heart and soul is missing now." If this is you, then you'll also be on the couch worrying about bills, the lack of finances and what the future holds but you have lost something even greater. Your job was not just a paycheck; it was your LIFE. You chose to make your career a high priority. Sickness has ripped it away and you are grieving.

People with chronic Lyme disease are forced to face this every day. Sometimes we willingly walk away from our jobs because our health is failing. Other times we're relieved of our duties because we can't keep up. Sometimes the parting is amicable; the employers support you for as long as possible but your illness interferes with job performance. Employers may go to great lengths to change workloads, give flexible schedules, allow extra days off and extend health insurance benefits, even if the person has gone to part-time. That's rare.

Unfortunately, chronically ill employees are usually forced to fight for that to which they're legally entitled. They try to continue normal work hours with failing bodies, compensating by taking copious notes, napping on their lunch hour and consuming loads of caffeine to battle fatigue. They stay late to finish work that now takes twice as long to complete or they bring work home. They struggle to fit in doctor's appointments, treatments, diets and medications without disrupting their work. They battle for benefits owed to them by law and pay exorbitant health insurance premiums. The greatest travesty of all is that employees can't be honest about being sick. If word leaks out that they're suffering from a chronic illness, it gets them an express ticket to the unemployment line.

Gone are the days where loyalty was the most important attribute to an employer. We no longer live in a society where we retire from a job after forty years and are thrown a huge retirement party. We can't count on the security of employers holding our spot while we're ill, wishing us well, checking our progress and welcoming us back upon recovery. It's ancient history for the company's health insurance to cover ALL medical expenses at no cost to us, simply because we are cherished employees and carry their insurance card. The burden of chronic illness now falls fully upon the individual and nothing is guaranteed when it comes to our future in the workplace.

As we agonize here in our beds, our physical state pales in comparison to the mental anguish we experience over how we'll rebuild our lives. The road to starting over is different for every chronically ill person. For those of us who have lost a beloved job, the pain is even more intense. It takes time, a great support system and a strong will to crawl our way back into the working world but it can be done.

There's no question that you are a different person now than before your life was turned upside down. You have just walked through the fires of hell and survived. You possess the power to reach your goals. Use this time of convalescence to heal your body and open your mind to new possibilities. Though you may not be able to return to the career you once loved, you still have much to offer this world. You've been given the opportunity to stop the frenetic pace of life and focus on what is important to you. Consider this a gift that not many people get. Learn from this time of chronic illness and use it as you move forward in creating your new life. Starting over may be the best thing that ever happened to you.

Regaining Your Sense Of Purpose (And Income) Online
By Louise Bibby

One of the most profound impacts chronic illness has upon our lives is the loss of sense of purpose, which ultimately leads to the loss of our sense of identity. This isn't just something I noticed in my own journey with chronic illness; research supports this.

I am passionate about empowering and encouraging others with chronic illness to discover or rediscover their purpose by following their passions, regardless of their physical circumstances. Thankfully, the opportunities available online for this are practically infinite!

I learned about online business in early 2013 by listening to Pat Flynn's Smart Passive Income podcast. Since then I've become a strong proponent for building passive income using blogs and other online methods. As loss of income is a major issue for those of us with chronic illness, I hope to be an example for using one's passion to gain a sense of purpose AND financial freedom.

Passive income involves some kind of action, often on-going, that can be done at your own pace which is a blessing for the chronically ill. Here are some ways you can earn income online while pursuing your passion:

1. Blogging and eBooks

Blogging and setting up your own website is a great, low-cost way to earn passive income. Attract others to your site by writing articles of interest. If you select topics for which you have a real passion and can write well, you can build an audience over time. The keys are to be patient, be consistent in writing content and get that content out to the appropriate audience – usually through social media.

How do you start blogging? I suggest signing up for a Wordpress.com or other free website to see if blogging is for you. Then start writing blogs about your passions. Seek out blogging podcasts, starting with Pat Flynn's Smart Passive Income (search for blogging in the podcast section). Also BecomeABlogger.com is a helpful podcast and site, as is Internet Business Mastery. Eventually you can buy a website on which to base your blog. I went with Bluehost for about $60 the first year, which includes the cost of the domain name.

To turn your writing into eBooks, I recommend signing up for Pat Flynn's newsletter, which gives you a bonus free eBook - eBooks the SMART Way. Also, I discovered a great site -AmyLynnAndrews.com - which has step-by-step blogs about writing and selling an eBook.

2. YouTube/Vlogging

If writing isn't your thing, you can always create a YouTube channel focused on topics you're passionate about. There are many blogs and podcasts out there to guide you on how to build online income this way. If you would like some guidance on finding resources, I'd be happy to help! Contact me at @GetUpNGoGuru on Twitter or via my Facebook page.

3. Affiliate Income

With affiliate marketing, you are rewarded as an affiliate for every customer you bring to the website of a designated business. When I learned about affiliate income, I got excited about its possibilities for earning money passively. The best tutorials on this topic can be found on Pat Flynn's Smart Passive Income podcast, including a 3-episode series on what affiliate income is and all the types out there. (If you are reading this on Kindle, see this page for all the links.)

My tips for earning through affiliate programs:

- If you're going to put affiliate ads on your site, make sure they look tasteful and don't clog your site up. I get put off when people have ads positioned randomly through their blog posts (via Google Adwords)!
- Don't spam. Use affiliate links where they are appropriate to your content and when they benefit your audience. Putting them up out of context on Twitter, Facebook or in emails will not win you any fans.
- Be genuine. I will only recommend something I have used myself or someone I really trust has recommended.

You can earn affiliate income with YouTube channels by putting links into your videos and/or the descriptions. Once again, be sure not to alienate your audience. Serving your audience needs to be your main priority to be a success in the long-term.

4. Ads on blogs/YouTube/podcasts

There are a range of ways you can put advertising on your blog/YouTube channel/podcast. You can sign up for Google Adwords. From my experience, they often look quite tacky on a blog and you need a lot of traffic to make any decent money.

With YouTube you can just tick a box to allow ads to come up before and during your videos. This is cleaner than Adwords because YouTubers can close the ads at a certain point. In-video ads are possible but I would limit that to what's relevant to your content – for instance, when reviewing a product.

5. So many opportunities, so little time and space!

There are thousands of websites dedicated to the topic of earning income online; I can't do justice to it all here. I'm happy to support you in any way I can to get you up and running, pursuing your passions and regaining your sense of purpose, while hopefully earning income from your toils.

(Editor's note: be sure to research your sources thoroughly and be discerning before committing to an online income opportunity.)

Art And Chronic Pain
By Nathalie Sheridan

Art - in particular, the latest craze for adult colouring books - has an enormous effect on improving health. Painting, drawing, doodling or colouring-in concentrates the mind, leaving no room for everyday stress. I find that, like reading, it slows my breathing down and I feel much calmer. With colouring-in or drawing, hand-to-eye co-ordination improves, too. I have discovered that even a short spell of immersing myself in art, perhaps only 20 minutes is enough to take my mind off my chronic pain, and all sufferers would agree that you need a break from pain now and then.

Research where you can find galleries and museums nearby so the next time you need a mental break, you'll know where to go! In many European countries, I've found that galleries have good accessibility for people with disabilities and mobility problems. Entrance fees for disabled people are reduced and entrance for caregivers who accompany you are often waived completely.

Whether you create art or enjoy other's creations, art is like a vacation for pain!

Finding My Joy Through A Lens
By *Anne Gaucher*
Aka "Lyme Lens"

I've loved art since middle school and began photography in high school, so it's been a long-time affair. In my photography, I like the way natural light hits things - lightning bolts, sunlight, sunset, sunbeams - any type of reflection of light and how it changes an image. I also tend to lean towards landscapes more than anything else. Even when I draw, I only use non-colored pencils because it's all about the light and shadows.

I prefer capturing a real moment in time with little-to-no manipulation. I don't like staged scenes, filters, artificial lighting, enhancements or computer graphics to alter a photograph. A great photographer can see instantly how common structures are manipulated by natural light and by using a simple camera with no special filters or lenses, they can capture an image that takes your breath away.

Before my illness, I would have loved to have been a journalist and war photographer. (I started college with a major in broadcast journalism.) We were on the verge of war and I wanted to report the news; to tell stories of troops from the front lines. Things just didn't work out that way.

Now, my photography reminds me that there is still life waiting to be lived. God has given me a gift of seeing light in a unique way. If I can take beautiful photographs and share them with someone who can no longer enjoy the outdoors then this is my new calling. Either way, I hope to recognize what HE has made and capture that moment for others to enjoy, even after I'm long gone.

Quotes About Passion And Purpose

My best tool for surviving chronic pain is my creativity, a true blessing. It helps me relax. Whenever I sketch, scrapbook, take photographs, or make jewelry, I forget the pain. It is much more tolerable while I am completely absorbed in a project.

– Katherine Dunn, jewelry maker

I wouldn't have found my calling if not for these illnesses. I've always loved Christian Hip-Hop, but never had the courage to record my own…The joy brought by writing a lyric that resonates with others, or finding the perfect instrumental, is indescribable. That's proof enough God is always working, even if I don't feel it.

– Becca Doss, songwriter

My first thought after I heard, "You have cancer," was of our daughter. My focus and goal became making her dream come true, and after much determination, I was finally able to say, "Dream Accomplished!" I can't describe the enormity of that moment or feeling. It was like a match lit a fire in my soul. I knew in my heart that even in my darkest hour, I was still capable of anything.

– Elizabeth Gross, author of <u>Dream Accomplished: A Story of Cancer, A Mother's Love & Taylor Swift</u>

I was laying in my bed one night and felt inspired to start "Spoonie Style Guide," my series on YouTube. Since I rarely leave my house and I can barely talk on the phone now, my major contact with others is through social media. I started my YouTube channel to inspire other people with chronic illness to live, optimize their energy, have fun and do it in style.

– Melanie Styles, YouTube video producer

Chapter 6
Grace and Warriorship:
Your Power to Affect Change

Blaze Your Beautiful Trail
By Grace Quantock

(Editor's note: This chapter was developed from Grace's globally-renowned TEDx Talk, "You're Not Broken, You're Breaking Boundaries.")

Every human will experience pain, grief, trauma and challenge of some kind. It can leave us feeling broken, different, outside, other.

We don't fit in and maybe never will - it hurts. What if it doesn't have to be this way?

I have been an outsider almost from the very beginning. A "freak" on many levels. Strangely small, strangely high-achieving, strangely surviving beyond the odds. I've got a rich yet eccentric background to which I've grown accustomed and deeply proud of over time, in spite of (and perhaps because of) the challenges and bullying I have faced.

Difference doesn't have to equal shame. I've never striven to "fit in" – a good thing, as my mother commented last week, as it would have been a losing battle from the start.

For years, I could pass as "normal" if I tried very hard. When I was 18, I got my first wheelchair and the differences became unmistakable.

Since then, people have approached me on the street, asked about my prognosis and cried upon hearing it. Others touched my legs to see if I was paralysed, put their hands on my head and prayed while I shopped and questioned me about my internal organs at bus stops.

I was tired of always being the "sick chick."

It was the first impression people got and one of the first things I was asked about. "What's wrong with you?" or, if we'd met before, "Aren't you better yet?" There was an ignorance and impatience in the questioning that implied I was not only imperfect but also a slow coach — that if I just worked harder, somehow, I should be able to "get back" to "100% normal."

The thing is, I felt it, too. A little bit at least. I fell into their way of thinking and judged myself. Convinced myself that I must somehow be in the wrong because they seemed so sure of themselves, while I just felt...confused.

My inaccurate self-perception and negative self-talk further played into all these judgements. I could only do that for so long.

It is all too easy in the culture which venerates perfection and power to see ourselves as broken. I have felt so tired. That bone-deep, dragging, exhausted ache from the pain of always feeling different.

What if we're not all outsiders? What if, instead, we are actually pioneers, radicals, change-makers and trailblazers?

I flipped my thinking. I embraced empowerment. I consciously tossed the feelings of inadequacy, grabbed hold of my own self-worth and did so while accepting my conditions. I didn't have to let my health be my identity, but I also didn't have to try to pass myself off as non-disabled. I can acknowledge my health, see my conditions...and carry on living anyway. Maybe not in the same way but I can still live life in my way.

I wasn't "the other," "the sick chick," odd or different. I was simply - and wonderfully! - me. The true trailblazing act of choosing to be myself in a world that always wants me to be something else. To opt out of all the given labels and create my own – "Trailblazer."

If I must live off the beaten track, I'll tread one of my own. My way. My path.

That takes courage.

How do we begin? How do we blaze our own trails and claim our liberation? Begin with yourself, your beliefs. Notice your language. Where are you blaming yourself? Does that guilt belong to you? If not, can you hand it back?

We call ourselves "wellness warriors," living with illness can feel like a battle to survive. To truly see and accept ourselves, we need to be graceful, too. To not be hard warriors all the time. To show ourselves compassion, kindness and love - and show our fellow warriors the same.

What happens if we view ourselves like a pioneer in training? What happens to our choices, thoughts and lives if we see them from the light of giving ourselves what we need to survive? How will supplying ourselves with the resources to thrive, in the situations in which we find ourselves, shift things? Let's find out together!

You aren't broken, you are a beautiful Trailblazer - going against the grain by choosing to see yourself as beautiful instead of broken, a pioneer instead of just poorly; empowered, instead of empty. Exercising your choice to redefine what it means to truly live with a health challenge.

Your empowerment in being different is liberating for every other misfit out there. Being a "misfit" can be a catalyst to forge an even greater destiny.

Maybe we are different. We can't help that. We can choose how we want to be different. We can work to handle life around us, holding onto ourselves and each other. We can opt to take what we have and live it in our own way, on our own terms.

We have the choice to be empowered, graceful warriors, blazing our own beautiful trails through the world.

Disease Is Dynamic; I Must Be Dynamic, Too
By Kari Ulrich

When I was diagnosed with a rare vascular disease called fibromuscular dysplasia (FMD), I relied on the internet to educate myself. Social media also gave me the ability to connect with patients around the world. I quickly realized becoming a patient advocate, using the internet, could not only change lives, it could save lives.

Being told you have a rare disease is devastating. Instinct takes over; I decided to fight. Like many empowered patients, I found both reliable and not-so-reliable sources on the web. I also noticed that patients like myself expressed two main concerns about their health care: first, their doctors did not take their symptoms seriously; second, many patients are frequently given misinformation or no information regarding their disease.

For me, this was a beginning of a long list of diagnoses, each with its own monitoring, treatment and prevention. My life and my family's lives changed at a rapid pace. I realized that I couldn't prevent dis-ease and preserve my health alone, nor could my family, friends and therapists give me all the support I needed. It takes a team of advocates.

The greatest support I've found comes from fellow patients and survivors - the "healers" that share our experience and have wisdom beyond physicians, family and friends. My team of healers comes from around the world and each person brings a fresh perspective to the conversation. They validate every fear, frustration, success and accomplishment we each experience and share knowledge from their own physicians to use for the betterment of our care. Connecting through social media has helped me in processing my experience and healing with my disease. I've felt less alone.

Social media allows us to connect with a community of healthcare professionals and patients 24/7. I was fortunate to meet a young girl through Facebook named Ashleigh, from South Africa, who has a rare form of FMD. Facebook became a significant tool in getting Ashleigh the proper medical care that she needed at the Cleveland Clinic. I was also able to help her family fundraise to pay for her care.

Social media is also critical in the world of rare and undiagnosed diseases for accurate and updated medical information. I've held Twitter chats that have benefited patients, educated medical professionals and connected with researchers.

In 2010, I co-founded a support group called Midwest Women's Vascular Advocates to support and educate those afflicted with my disease and other non-inflammatory vascular diseases. We utilized Facebook and a website to connect with others. Locally we held support group meetings and drew patients from out of state. Our advocate group became family; we laughed, cried, celebrated our victories and mourned our losses.

Being an organization lead by patients can take its toll. As our leadership's health changed, it became difficult to carry on the task of continuing formally as a group. Today we still enjoy a great sense of belonging and know we can lean on each other whenever the need arises.

Patient advocates are revolutionizing health care. They take a road less traveled to make the path easier for others and lay the foundation of open communication within the health care community. I believe it goes beyond caring for the human being; there is a compassion in the advocate's soul that cannot be defined by words.

When a health care provider has, on average, 10 minutes' time devoted to patient care including the physical exam and documentation, it does not leave enough time for active listening. WE LISTEN; we become a voice for many who are too exhausted by the health care system to speak for themselves.

Patient advocates listen in several ways that physicians do not. We blog and make known how our daily life is affected by disease, enable other patients to interact and give each other an opportunity to listen to our experiences. We are active users of Facebook and Twitter, helpful tools for active listeners. We let patients process and work through their disease. We develop relationships through social media that spill over to more traditional ways of communicating ie. the telephone! My long-distance bill has dramatically increased over the years from calls with patients across the United States and as far as South Africa. Each phone call ends with the words, "Thank you for taking the time to listen."

The opportunities for patient advocates are unlimited. I was honored to participate in Mayo Clinic's Social Media Summit. Participation encouraged me to open doors, both locally and globally. The world of health care in social media is branching out in many directions from support and advocacy to education and research.

Why do we advocate and take the time to listen? Advocates gain wisdom from listening; we're educational sponges trying to soak up and process information, then voice this information to others. We get our energy from connecting. We don't let our disease define us but rather we take control of our lives in a proactive way that also serves others. Our reward is in seeing relationships built and communication opening within the health care community. We are partners in the health care team that are making the future better for us all.

Twitter: @FMDGirl

LinkedIn: www.linkedin.com/in/kariulrichrn

Blog: fibromusculardysplasia.blogspot.com

Facebook: www.facebook.com/FMDGirl

The Therapeutic Power Of Creative Expression
By Mary Pettigrew

Sometime around 2010, I became an avid user of social media (specifically Twitter) to learn and interact with poets, writers, people with multiple sclerosis (MS) and other chronic illnesses. In fact, Twitter is where I first became involved with Pajama Daze and met lovely people living with chronic illness who had the same creative passion that I have. I've remained close friends with many people from that group to this day.

I continued to meet people and explore the opportunities social media had to offer, attending various live chats with topics ranging from health issues to screenwriting and blogging. SpoonieChat was (and still is) an inspirational group of people living with chronic illness and I want to thank them for their role and guidance which inspired me to reinvent and rediscover myself. I found a purpose and passion through creative expression I never knew existed. There it was, hidden within me, buried under the covers of my bed. I learned so much from people who were just like myself. Creative individuals who could no longer work, who were frequently confined to their bed, yet still had something special to offer!

Creative writing became my focus; it still is. I couldn't wait to share my words with others and my hope was to inspire someone, at least one person, into exploring ways to express themselves creatively in ANY form or fashion!

Towards the end of 2013, the MS and chronic illness online communities I had grown to love had expanded to the point I could no longer keep up with them on a regular basis. Too many people were trying to join in various chains of conversation which became cumbersome. With Twitter, if numerous people are chatting and chiming in at once, there is NO ROOM to converse. This is frustrating for so many people.

After brainstorming and proposing ideas to online friends, we decided to try something new; to move beyond my own personal account and open a new account specifically for the MS community. Eventually a team of administrators came together, Carolyn Palmer (a fellow MSer) partnered with me in all our projects and MSpals was born.

Besides our main Twitter, Facebook and Pinterest accounts, I started a poetry account called Chronically Creative for people with chronic illness to post poetry on Twitter, based on a daily word prompt that I provide. I had started writing and participating in other daily writing prompt groups and the therapy was MAGICAL! To this day, our prompt group is considered one of the favorite poetry prompt groups on Twitter. Darla Vaughan is my partner for this group as it grows. We all work hard to interact and be present. There are apps available to automatically schedule posts or tweets, weeks or even months in advance, which makes things easier.

MSpals added several special interest groups on Facebook, including a "creative expression" group. This group is not limited to creative writing; it's for all kinds of artistic works and activities. As MSpals grew, positive word of mouth spread, encouraging people to join. Other groups became attracted to our work and we partner with many to ensure a healthy relationship. They help us, we help them!

With the assistance of other like-minded friends, MSpals evolved into something unique and unlike any other group found on social media. At the time of this writing, MSpals maintains a combined membership with well over 8000 people. The National MS Society took notice of MSpals and the "power of online connecting" and in 2014, interviewed me and a few of my administrators for an article in their quarterly publication, Momentum Magazine. (The same magazine interviewed me and others living with MS about the power of "art and MS" a couple years earlier.)

When we can, Carolyn and I attend local support groups together and often connect with our local NMSS chapter. I have served on the steering committee for an annual fundraiser for the last three years. No matter what I do or where I am, I do my best to promote and tell the story of MSpals. Our members are doing the same – globally!

In March 2016, I created another poetry group on Facebook collaborating with three other people with disabilities. This new group is not MS specific but for people with ALL disabilities and chronic illness to write and share poetry and prose.

The therapeutic power of creative expression is something to behold and the possibilities are endless!

Burning Nights
By *Victoria Abbott-Fleming*

After I was diagnosed with complex regional pain syndrome (CRPS) for a second time in 2014, my husband and I decided life was precious and short, so we created an awareness and support website for other CRPS sufferers. We designed a forum to chat, rant and swap tips with others as well as regular blogs, newsletters, an online shop and a page with the latest information and research about the condition. I named it "Burning Nights CRPS Support" because the burning pain for me tends to worsen at night when we begin relaxing and calming down after the day's events. The website and social media campaigns finally went live in August 2014 at www.burningnightscrps.org.

There hadn't been anything like this in the UK since 2008 so I wanted to start getting things going right away. I began researching every aspect of CRPS so our website would be based on solid evidence. I was very determined to get it off the ground and make sure it worked so people with CRPS, not just from the UK but worldwide, had a place to connect with others who understood what they were going through. It was also a space for loved ones, caregivers, families and friends to chat and learn how to cope with living with a CRPS sufferer.

Unfortunately, as Burning Nights started to move forward at the end of November, the skin on my left CRPS leg started to break down and ulcerate just like it had done on the right. I couldn't believe it, not again! Within one week the front and side of my leg had completely opened with ulcers and the weeping started AGAIN! My second above-knee amputation occurred on the 15th of December 2014. I was more worried about the followers on Burning Nights and how they were doing than I was about my own recovery from surgery.

I am thrilled at how sufferers have taken to Burning Nights on the forum, website and social media! We seem to be going from strength to strength. We took on trustees and more volunteers for social media as I couldn't deal with it all myself. After 7 months of application, Burning Nights CRPS Support became a UK registered charity dedicated to raising awareness and supporting anyone affected by CRPS, whether they are sufferers, caregivers, family members, loved ones or friends. CRPS doesn't just affect the sufferer; it affects all those around them.

We do fundraising as a group and others arrange fundraising events, including sponsored events, swimming events, summer BBQs and more. We have an annual conference in a hotel with professional medical speakers, as well as CRPS sufferers and caregivers to recount their journeys through life with complex regional pain syndrome. We offer local support groups which are going well. Since January 2016, we've operated a telephone line for information, help and support for anyone with this condition or their families, friends and caregivers. The phone line is answered by fellow CRPS sufferers. We are not medically trained so we can cannot offer medical advice or diagnoses but we are there to support and offer help, answer questions and provide information about the condition.

Our small online shop offers CRPS awareness leaflets, postcards and bookmarks, as well as medical alert USBs for chronic conditions or CRPS. We have promotional items such as a pen, wristband, pet bandana and enamel pin badge. Our products are posted around the world; we accept the UK pound and other currencies.

As a charity, we also arrange seminars, awareness training and talks for healthcare and legal professionals. We eventually aim to have CRPS support groups around the entire UK so anyone affected by the condition has local support. We ultimately hope to have a board of medical professionals, not only to support us as a charity but to help organise hospital protocols. Our goal is that when someone presents at a hospital with CRPS symptoms, the medical staff will be able to evaluate the condition of the patient and then get them seen by either the pain clinic or pain specialist to determine whether the patient has CRPS.

Our first year as a registered CRPS charity was amazing, as not only were our support groups, conferences and fundraisers well-received but we were awarded 'Charity of the Year' by Aspire Magazine, which is an amazing feat for a first-year charity. Also, I was awarded the 'Crystal Trophy for Inspirational Woman of the Year!' I am still a little speechless but very honoured to be awarded this amazing accolade. I accepted the award on behalf of all the CRPS sufferers and their families affected by this horrific condition.

I'm grateful to all who have supported Burning Nights CRPS Support, our trustees and volunteers.

Recommended Reading

Memoirs

Yvonne deSousa, <u>MS Madness! A "Giggle More, Cry Less" Story of Multiple Sclerosis</u>. East Bridgewater, Massachusetts: SDP Publishing. 2013.

Cynthia Toussaint with Linden Gross, <u>Battle for Grace: A Memoir of Pain, Redemption and Impossible Love</u>. Self-published. 2013.

Cindy Yee Kong, <u>The Eyes of the Lion: A Memoir</u>. Bloomington, Indiana: Abbott Press. 2013.

Dan and Jennifer Digmann, <u>Despite MS, to Spite MS: One couple facing the challenges of life and Multiple Sclerosis</u>. Mount Pleasant, Michigan: Magee Press. 2011.

Elizabeth Gross, <u>Dream Accomplished: A Story of Cancer, a Mother's Love and Taylor Swift</u>. Self-published. 2015.

Dennis Maione, <u>What I Learned from Cancer</u>. Self-published. 2014.

Suzanne Robins, <u>Faulty Wiring: Living with Invisible MS</u>. Self-published. 2013.

Living with Chronic Illness

Michael Fernandez, <u>One Man's Chronic Pain: Poetry from the Heart</u>. Self-published. 2013.

Lene Andersen, <u>Chronic Christmas: Surviving the Holidays with a Chronic Illness</u>. Two North Books. 2016.

Lene Andersen, <u>Your Life with Rheumatoid Arthritis: Tools for Managing Treatment, Side Effects and Pain</u>. Two North Books. 2013.

Lene Andersen, <u>7 Facets: A Meditation on Pain</u>. Two North Books. 2013.

Toni Bernhard, <u>How to Live Well with Chronic Pain and Illness: A Mindful Guide</u>. Somerville, Massachusetts: Wisdom Publications. 2015.

Toni Bernhard, <u>How to Be Sick: A Buddhist-Inspired Guide for the Chronically Ill and Their Caregivers</u>. Somerville, Massachusets. Wisdom Publications. 2010.

Stephanie Davis, Through the Eye of Migraine. Tampa/Clearwater: Bouncy Boxer Media. 2013.

Richard Cheu, Living Well with Chronic Illness: A Practical and Spiritual Guide. Indianapolis, Indiana: Dog Ear Publishing. 2013.

Elizabeth Turp, Chronic Fatigue Syndrome/ME: Support for Family and Friends. London, United Kingdom and Philadelphia, Pennsylvania: Jessica Kingsley Publishers. 2011.

Shoosh Lettick Crotzer, Yoga for Fibromyalgia: Move, Breathe, and Relax to Improve Your Quality of Life. Berkley, California: Rodmell Press. 2008.

Jon Kabat-Zinn, Ph.D., Full Catastrophe Living: Using the Wisdom of Your Body and Mind to Face Stress, Pain, and Illness (Revised Edition). New York, New York: Bantam Books. 2013.

Mary C. Earle, Broken Body, Healing Spirit: Lectio Divina and Living with Illness. Harrisburg, Pennsylvania: Morehouse Publishing. 2003.

Wayne and Sherri Connell, "But You LOOK Good": How to Encourage and Understand People Living with Illness and Pain. Parker, Colorado: Indivisible Disabilities Association. 2013.

Trixie Whitmore, Toxic Chemical-Free Living and Recovering from ME/CFS. Birchgrove, New South Wales, Australia: Sally Milner Publishing Pty Ltd. 1990.

Richard Thomas with Consultant Dr. Tim Nash, Alternative Answers to Pain: All your options, conventional and complementary, for beating the problem of chronic pain. London, United Kingdom: New Burlington Books. 1999.

Laurie Edwards, Life Disrupted: Getting Real About Chronic Illness in Your Twenties and Thirties. New York, New York: Walker Publishing Company, Inc. 2008.

Tia Borkowski, It's All In Your Head & Other Things I've Been Told: Poems about chronic illness, mental illness, and life & love with both. Self-published. 2018.

Howard Schubiner, MD, Unlearn Your Pain: A 28-Day Process to Reprogram Your Brain. Pleasant Ridge, WI: Mind Body Publishing, 2016.

Getting Through Tough Times

Tom Ingrassia and Jared Chrudimsky, <u>One Door Closes: Overcoming Adversity by Following Your Dreams</u>. USA: MotivAct Publishing. 2013.

Frances Bingham, <u>How to Improve Your Life in 15 Minutes a Day</u>. (journal) Self-published. 2016.

Amy Newmark, <u>Chicken Soup for the Soul: Finding Your Inner Strength – 101 Empowering Stories of Resilience, Positive Thinking, and Overcoming Challenges</u>. Cos Cob, Connecticut: Chicken Soup for the Soul Publishing. 2014.

Lisa and Franco Esile, <u>Whose Mind Is It Anyway? Get Out of Your Head and Into Your Life</u>. New York, New York: Tarcher Perigree. 2016.

Maggie Oman Shannon, <u>Prayers for Healing: 365 Blessings, Poems, & Meditations from Around the World</u>. York Beach, Maine: Conari Press. 2000.

Taking Care of Your Whole Health

Jennifer Mulder, "How to Create Your Own Action Plan for Recovery: A step-by-step guide on rebuilding your health after illness or injury." Self-published Ebook. 2017. Health Sessions (www.healthsessions.com)

Martine Ehrenclou, <u>The Take Charge Patient: How You Can Get the Best Medical Care</u>. Santa Monica, California: Lemon Grove Press LLC. 2012.

Martine Ehrenclou, <u>Critical Conditions: The Essential Hospital Guide to Get Your Loved One Out Alive</u>. Santa Monica, California: Lemon Grove Press LLC. 2008.

Jerome Groopman, M.D., <u>How Doctors Think</u>. New York, New York: Mariner Books. 2008.

Bill Moyers, <u>Healing and the Mind</u>. New York, New York: Doubleday. 1993.

Andrew Weil, M.D., <u>Eating Well for Optimum Health: The Essential Guide to Food, Diet, and Nutrition</u>. New York, New York: Albert A. Knopf. 2000.

Caregiving

Nannette J. David, Ph.D., <u>The ABCs of Caregiving: Words to Inspire You</u>. Bellingham, Washington: House of Harmony Press. 2013.

Angil Tarach-Ritchey, <u>Behind the Old Face: Aging in America and the Coming Elder Boom</u>. Sonoma, California: DreamSculpt Media, Inc. 2012.

Epilogue

As I put the finishing touches on this book, I must acknowledge what has happened in my life in the past year. Last August, after losing my apartment of 8 years, I moved in temporarily with a friend until I was able to find a suitable place to live. I finally found my slice of heaven in the mountains of Peterborough, New Hampshire, just 45 minutes from family and an hour and a half from my medical care in Boston. I had to downsize dramatically, which was an elongated process of sorting and selling and giving away at both ends of the move. I arrived in a new town that held promise for a delightful new chapter in my life.

On June 3rd, the day I moved in, I received a call from my brother-in-law in Pennsylvania. My sister, Leslie, who had MS and various other painful conditions for many years, had been deteriorating both physically and mentally, as I had witnessed in our phone calls and emails. She had not gotten the help she needed at home nor in the medical system. Many times when I offered help, it was pushed away. On June 2nd, 2018, her husband drove her to the doctor because of intense pain. That day my sister became another statistic: she was refused pain medication because of the "opioid crisis." She went home, closed the bedroom door and took her own life.

Two weeks later, I was diagnosed with Stage 1 invasive ductal carcinoma, an intermediately aggressive breast cancer (ER-, PR-, HER2+). I was put on a chemotherapy regimen which included Taxol and targeted drugs, followed by surgery, radiation and nine months of continued targeted drugs. Any less and my chance of survival would diminish. I am happy to report that my tumor shrank to half its size, it was removed with clean margins and all six lymph nodes were clear. I am kicking this cancer to the curb!

And then there was my back. I have had occasional back and neck pain for most of my life. But enduring two moves in the past year wreaked havoc on my spine. Pain became increasingly serious after my second month in New Hampshire. The MRIs showed bulging and herniated disks throughout my spine, impinging on nerves and the spinal cord. The disc at L1-L2 posed a significant problem with back pain and the use of my right leg. Two weeks before my breast cancer surgery, I had successful surgery on the worse disc and regained comfort and function!

How did I handle all the recent tragedy, challenges and change? I wept, I got angry, I denied, I blamed, I floundered. But I didn't stay there. Once the emotions were out, there was room for faith, hope, love, acceptance, humor and resilience to take over. Again, any less and my chance of survival would diminish! All the challenges and chronic illness that I have dealt with previously taught me much about handling this onslaught of crises and gave me strength to forge through it. And I must give credit to the books about chronic illness that I reviewed for my website, pajamadaze.com. I learned valuable lessons from each and every one of them.

I grieved for my sister while she was still alive and suffering. Every day was physical and mental torture for her. Had she embraced the help I offered, had her medical practitioners been proactive, compassionate and supportive, and had she had assistance at home to improve her quality of life, her story may have ended differently. We will never know. I feel deeply sad now that she is gone, yet relieved for her. She has been released from her hell.

I use my infusion days at the hospital as special self-care time. I wrap myself in a prayer shawl that a loving friend gave to me, listen to Enya and color in beautiful intricate coloring books, eating grapes and the lunch they offer. These are "me days" that I actually enjoy. I picture the drugs going into my body and gobbling up all the cancer nasties. I did lose my hair but was never very ill from the chemo. Perhaps embracing the process as well as healthy habits have a positive impact on the effects and success of treatment.

Meanwhile, I try to take advantage of the free and inexpensive opportunities to entertain and enrich my life in my new town. I made a friend who is a harpist; she is teaching me to play the bowed psaltery so we can play music for shut-ins and nursing homes (it is very easy; I play it by ear). I have enjoyed free concerts and lectures, art galleries and funky outdoor cafes where I can watch the world go by. When able, I walk through the tended gardens of the downtown, or down my country road where there is always something to discover. One day, I hope to embark on my maiden voyage in a kayak across Cunningham Pond with my best friend from childhood, Carole. Life is opening up with new possibilities full of creativity and joy.

I am looking ahead to when my cancer journey is complete, hopefully at the end of Summer 2019. It has been a tough year, but I remain grateful for all the blessings in my life, hopeful for the future and continue to marvel at the little miracles that appear every day.

If we can be grateful for even one blessing each day, we're living a good life.

Cameron B. Auxer, November 21, 2018

Appendix

The Take-Charge Patient's Toolkit
By Martine Ehrenclou

(Reprinted with the author's permission)

Health Summary

Complete this form before you see a doctor about a medical problem. Take it with you to the office visit.

(Editor's note: Bring a current list of medications, as well.)

Full name	Date of birth
Home Phone	Cell phone
Physician's name/contact #	Emergency contact/contact #

REASON FOR THIS VISIT	Date __ /__ /__

My top 5 questions for the doctor:

Describe your symptoms. Use diagrams at right to show where they are located.

When did symptoms start? How often are they present?	How severe is pain on a scale from 1-10?

What makes them worse or better? If you had symptoms before, how were they treated and how successful was the treatment?

Health History

Complete this form & keep it in your health file at home.
Take a copy with you to new medical providers.

Full name	Date of birth
Home phone	Cell phone
Physician's name and contact information	Emergency contact info

MAJOR SURGERIES

Date	Description	Surgeon's name/contact info
Date	Description	Surgeon's name/contact info

SIGNIFICANT PROCEDURES AND TESTS

Date	Description	Doctor's name/contact info
	Results	
Date	Description	Doctor's name/contact info
	Results	

\

Medical Conditions and Illnesses

Date of onset	Description	Treatment & results
Date of onset	Description	Treatment & results
Date of onset	Description	Treatment & results

Questions To Ask Before You Select A New Doctor

- Does the doctor take my health insurance?

- Is the doctor board-certified in his/her specialty?

- Is the doctor affiliated with the hospital of my choice?

- How long does it usually take to get a routine appointment?

- How long does it take to get a sick appointment?

- How much time does the doctor usually spend with a patient?

- Is the doctor's office open when I am available to go? Ask about evening or Saturday appointments.

- Does the doctor's practice use a website for appointments, education or advice?

- Does the doctor have a nurse practitioner or physician's assistant?

Questions To Ask Yourself About Your Symptoms

- When did I first begin experiencing symptoms?

- When do I most notice the symptoms?

- How severe are my symptoms?

- Does anything make the symptoms worse or better?

- Have my symptoms changed over time?

- Where on or in my body are the symptoms located?

- Is there pain related to my symptoms?

- Were the symptoms or pain first triggered by a physical event?

- What have I tried to alleviate the symptoms?

- What do I think is causing my symptoms or associated pain?

Questions To Ask Your Doctor About Your Diagnosis And Treatment Plan

- What is my diagnosis?

- Where can I find information about my diagnosis?

- Do you have information you can give me?

- Are there any other possible diagnoses for my condition?

- What is my treatment plan?

- If you aren't confident or comfortable with the proposed treatment plan, ask the following: Are there alternatives to this treatment plan?

- How long do you think it will take for me to recover?

- Are there tests and procedures I need to have done?

- What changes do I need to make to support my recovery?

- Do I need another appointment with you?

- Do I feel comfortable with my diagnosis and treatment plan, or do I need a second opinion?

Questions To Ask About Medications

- What is the name of the medication you prescribed for me? (Ask for brand and generic names.) Spell it for me (many drugs sound the same).

- Does it matter whether I take the brand-name or generic version of this medication? Why?

- What is the dosage and how many times a day do I need to take it? What is the maximum dosage?

- How long will I be on the medication? When will it start to work?

- Why am I taking this medication? For what condition?

- Do I need to take this medication with or without food/milk or at any particular time of day?

- Are there any side effects to this medication? Can I drive? Can I drink alcohol?

- Can this medication interact with any of my other medications? Birth control pills?

Questions To Ask Your Doctor About Tests And Procedures

- Do I need to get copies of test results or reports from other doctors such as blood work, MRI, CT scan? (If so, keep a copy for yourself and get one for your medical provider. Keep your copy in your health file at home. You never know when you may need it.)

- What is the procedure or test that you are recommending?

- What are you looking for with this procedure/test?

- How long will it take?

- Do I have to prepare for this procedure/test? Fasting? Don't take certain meds?

- What are the risks and benefits to this procedure/test?

- Are there any side effects?

- Is this procedure/test covered by my health insurance?

- Will I be able to drive home after this procedure/test?

- Do I need to have someone drive me to the procedure/test? Stay at home with me after?

- Will I be able to go back to work right after the procedure/test? Recovery time after?

- Will there be pain or discomfort with the procedure/test? Will I be medicated?

- Do I feel comfortable with this procedure/test or do I need a second opinion?

- How many have you done? Any serious complications? (Typically asked for surgical procedures but can apply to biopsies)

Questions To Ask Your Doctor About A Surgery

- What is the surgery you want to perform?

- Is the hospital or surgery center covered by my health insurance?

- Is the anesthesiologist's fee covered by my health insurance?

- Do you have informational materials you can give me about this type of surgery?

- How many of these surgeries have you performed?

- What will the surgery do for me? What would happen if I didn't go through with this surgery?

- What are the risks to this type of surgery?

- Will the surgery be performed in the hospital or in a surgery center?

- What will my recovery be like? Please describe my after-care.

- Will I be in pain after the surgery? How do you treat pain?

- Will I need someone to help with my care after the surgery? To what extent?

- Do I feel comfortable with having this surgery or do I need a second opinion?

- How long will I be out of work, if at all? Will I have other restrictions ie. sports, driving, lifting?

Questions To Answer After Visiting My Medical Provider

- Did I feel comfortable with my medical provider? If not, list reasons.

- Did I get all of my questions answered? If not, list here.

- Do I need more information about what my medical provider shared with me? List here.

- What is my plan if I need more information? Do research? Call the doctor?

- What do I need to do now? Example: new treatment plan, modify current treatment plan, have a test or procedure or surgery etc.

- How was the office staff? Courteous? Was office clean? Was my privacy respected?

Questions To Ask Your Health Insurance Provider

- Do I have a co-pay? If so, how much is it?

- What is my deductible?

- What is my premium?

- Do I have co-insurance?

- Which medical providers does my insurance plan allow me to see?

- Which hospitals, clinics or surgery centers does my insurance plan allow me to use?

- Am I currently seeing in-network providers? How much do out-of-network providers cost?

- Will my health insurance pay anything if I see doctors who do not take insurance?

- Does my plan cover specific needs (specialist, vision, dental, chemotherapy, etc.)?

- Does my plan cover prescription medications?

- Does my health insurance cover nurse practitioners and physician's assistants?

- Does my plan cover acupuncture, physical therapy and other therapies?

- Does my plan cover me if I travel outside of my state/country?

- If I have primary and secondary insurance, do I understand what each covers?

- Does my plan cover any nursing home care, rehab facility admissions or hospice care?

My Medication Safety Checklist

- What is the name and dosage of the medication my medical provider prescribed? Check spelling.

- Why am I taking this medication?

- How do I take this medication? For example, with food, without food, time of day.

- What are the brand and generic names of this medication? (This is so you can match it to the medication you receive from your pharmacy.)

- Did I review the prescription in the doctor's office? Do I have refills?

- Did I look at the medication I received from my pharmacy? Check who it is for. Check the medication itself—do you recognize it? If not, call your pharmacy to make sure it's correct. (Editor's note: count pills to be sure you weren't shorted.)

- Do I need to set up an appointment to meet with my pharmacist?

- Do I need help managing my medications?

- Have I explored my options to get help to manage my medications? If not, ask your pharmacist for assistance.

- Have I created a list of all my medications? Carry it with you in wallet or purse. Update frequently.

- Have I considered using only one pharmacy? Highly recommended. Write name and phone # on med list.

- Do I need to set up timers to alert me to take my medications?

- Have I provided a list of my medication allergies to my physicians, other medical professionals and pharmacist? Do I need to consider a medical alert bracelet due to severe drug allergies?

Patient Safety Checklist

- Am I prepared for each doctor/medical provider with copies of pertinent test results, health summary, list of current medications, list of symptoms, questions for my medical provider and top three medical concerns? Do I have a list of questions?

- Did I research my diagnosis?

- Did I ask my doctor if there could be other possible diagnoses?

- Do I know my family medical history such as medical conditions or diseases my parents or siblings have? Have I shared this information with my medical provider?

- Did I create my own list of medications and their dosages, over-the-counter medications, herbs and supplements and shared that list with each medical provider I see?

- Did I follow up on my test results?

- Did I ask what my test results mean?

- Did I ask for my tests to be repeated?

- Have I enlisted support from loved ones?

- Do I need an advocate?

- Do I need a second opinion from a doctor who is affiliated with a respected medical school?

- Can I have a copy of my test results so I can review them again and keep them in my home file?

Your Medical ID Card

As a take-charge patient, you must create a medical ID card, one of the most important tools in your toolkit. Copy and print the card on the next page, cut it out, fill it out, and carry it with you at all times. Create a new one whenever there are changes. Medical apps for your information are great but you need this as a backup in case your medical app or smartphone cannot be found.

- Your medical ID card should contain the following information:
- Your full name.
- Your primary care physician's name and contact information or the name of any other medical professional who manages your care. This is the person you see the most for your primary care.
- Your current medical conditions, medications and their dosages, over-the-counter medications, including herbs and supplements, and allergies to medications. Your pharmacy name and phone #.
- Emergency contact names and phone numbers. List the person you want to be called if you have a medical emergency.

MEDICAL INFORMATION

Patient Name:

Home Address:

PCP:

Other Specialists Currently Seeing:

Current Medications:

Allergies to Medications:

Fold

Current Medical Conditions:

Current Diagnoses:

Emergency Contacts-

Spouse or Partner:

Friend or Family Member:

Caregiver if Applicable:

Preferred Hospital:

Health Insurance:

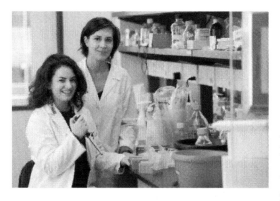

Benaroya Research Institute

By purchasing this book, you have helped to fund vital research into autoimmune disease at Benaroya Research Institute in Seattle, Washington.

Benaroya Research Institute at Virginia Mason Hospital and Medical Center (BRI) is committed to finding causes and cures for autoimmune diseases such as type 1 diabetes, rheumatoid arthritis, inflammatory bowel disease and multiple sclerosis. Our research is dedicated to predicting, preventing, halting, treating and ultimately eliminating these lifelong, chronic diseases.

An internationally-recognized medical research institute, located in Seattle, BRI accelerates discovery through laboratory breakthroughs in immunology that are then translated to clinical therapies.

BRI is involved in significant collaborative initiatives with industry, academia and government entities and leads the NIH funded Immune Tolerance Network, Type 1 Diabetes TrialNet and other major cooperative research programs resulting in worldwide scope and impact.

The unique way BRI works:

Discovery starts in the laboratory. One of the unique qualities of BRI is the close integration of three types of medical research—laboratory research, translational research and clinical research—to improve people's lives.

Translational Research and Biorepositories. Translational research is the link between laboratory research and clinical research, built upon an exchange of materials and information between these two disciplines.

Clinical Trials Bring Research Results to Patients. Clinical research studies involve individuals who volunteer to participate in new medical approaches not available outside the clinical trial setting.

Prevention of Diseases. One of the important lessons learned in BRI's quest to diagnose, better treat and cure autoimmune diseases is that earlier intervention is better than later intervention.

A Vision of Personalized Medicine. Immunology research is driving toward individualized treatment for each person with autoimmune and immune-mediated diseases.

Proceeds from this book support BRI's vital resources to test unfunded new ideas and theories on how to fight autoimmune diseases such as type 1 diabetes, multiple sclerosis, arthritis and other diseases. If you wish to make further donations, or to learn more, please visit BenaroyaResearch.org.